Federal Policy
toward
Mental Retardation
and
Developmental Disabilities

Federal Policy
toward
Mental Retardation
and
Developmental Disabilities

by

David Braddock, Ph.D.
Associate Professor of Community Health Sciences
School of Public Health
and
Institute for the Study of Developmental Disabilities
The University of Illinois at Chicago

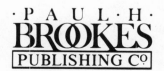

·P A U L·H·
BROOKES
PUBLISHING C?

Baltimore · London

Paul H. Brookes Publishing Co.
Post Office Box 10624
Baltimore, MD 21285-0624

Typeset by The Composing Room, Grand Rapids, Michigan.
Manufactured in the United States of America by
The Maple Press Company, York, Pennsylvania.

Library of Congress Cataloging-in-Publication Data

Braddock, David L.
   Federal policy toward mental retardation and developmental disabilities.

   Bibliography: p.
   Includes index.
   1. Mental retardation—Government policy—United States. 2. Developmental
disabilities—Government policy—United States. I. Title. [DNLM: 1. Child
Development Disorders—United States—legislation. 2. Handicapped—United
States—legislation. 3. Mental Retardation—United States—legislation. WS 33
AA1 B7f]
RC570.5.U6B73 1987   362.3'56'0973   86-11288
ISBN 0-933716-66-4

Contents

Listing of Tables and Figures By Chapter

Foreword

WHEN DAVID BRADDOCK invited me to prepare the foreword to this book, I said that I would be honored to do so. This book is the single most useful document about federal government policy toward mental retardation and developmental disabilities produced in the 28 years that I have served in the United States Congress. Its preparation was a formidable task and the author has carried it out with great depth and objectivity.

Although the primary focus of the book is on mental retardation and developmental disabilities policy, a great deal of information is presented on the history and accomplishments of federal programs pertaining to all disabilities. There is, for example, considerable detail on the financial and programmatic structure of federal special education, vocational rehabilitation, and public health programs. As a reference document alone, professionals in all facets of the disability field are going to want to have this volume in their libraries. It is essential reading for anyone interested in the federal government's important and changing role in the lives of 36 million Americans with disabilities.

Thirteen years ago, I began my service on the Senate Finance Committee, and beginning in 1980, I had the privilege of chairing that committee as it faced the challenges of financing the nation's health care. Each day it is becoming more apparent that we must begin shifting our primary focus from the acute health care market to the long-term health care market. Changing demographics have made long-term care spending the fastest growing segment of the U.S. health care industry. Average annual increases in our national expenditures for nursing home care, for example, consistently exceed the average for all other expenditures, including hospital care.

Today, responsibility for long-term care services is shared almost equally by the public and private sectors. Public responsibility rests mainly with the Medicaid program, which pays about 56% of our nation's nursing home bill. But the remainder of this bill, over $11 billion, comes directly from the pockets of patients and their families. Private insurance plays almost no role in the financing of long-term care, nor does Medicare, which has only limited provisions for post-hospital skilled nursing or rehabilitative care. Slowing the growth of long-term care expenditures—perhaps through a prospective payment system—and agreeing on the mix of public and private fiscal responsibility in this area are issues that will require further analysis and discussion.

So too, will the issue of locus of care. As Dr. Braddock points out, most long-term care services are now being provided in costly institutions. Less than one-quarter of our public long-term care expenditures pay for services delivered within the home or community. A redirection of this funding pattern is long overdue. Congress recently acted to allow states significantly greater flexibility in the development of home and community-based long-term care services. The response from the states has been enthusiastic. Creative and cost-effective programs are springing up from Maine to California and everywhere in between.

The continued escalation of the cost of health care needs to be examined in further depth so that a solution or solutions can be adopted that supports those who need our assistance—the poor, the elderly, and the disabled—and simultaneously maintains a system that provides the highest quality of care in the world. In 1984, health expenditures in the United States approached $400 billion—about 11% of the nation's gross national product, the highest such share in history.

Twenty-five years ago, health care expenditures constituted only 5% of the gross national product. The increase in medical costs in 1984 was also about twice the general rate of inflation.

Obviously, we live in a time of fiscal austerity. The federal budget is under seige to some hard economic realities. The federal government itself is trying to restore the historic concept of federalism before the foundation of American self-rule is smothered beneath Washington's deficits, Washington's rules, Washington's regulations, and Washington's smug conviction that it knows best.

The demands on our dollars have never been greater. But that does not mean any diminution in the needs of the disabled. What is just in a time of heavy spending remains equally just in a time of belt-tightening. Fortunately, I can report that programs for the disabled through Fiscal Year 1986, by and large, have escaped the budgetary ax. I see no desire in the future for a major retreat from the commitment of recent years, even notwithstanding the recent enactment of the Gramm-Rudman-Hollings legislation. If necessary, Congress must seriously consider adopting revenue enhancement measures as well as terminate certain inefficient government programs.

I see a future with a far greater reliance on partnerships between government and private industry. Government no longer has all the answers or the available resources to cope with the diversity of problems and needs within our society. Only by harnessing the energies and talents of all sectors of America can we successfully restore both human dignity and self-reliance to the lives of Americans with disabilities.

As this book so capably documents, we have come a long way. We still have a long distance to go. But we have a clear and worthy goal: to reduce the growing costs of disability in the United States, and to enable more persons with disabilities to lead productive lives through increased work opportunities, while providing benefits for those who cannot work. This will make a better America not only for our citizens with disabilities, but for all citizens.

Senator Bob Dole
U.S. Senate Majority Leader

Preface

FOR ANYONE INTERESTED in the history of public policy toward people with mental retardation and developmental disabilities in the United States, the first riffle through the pages of this book can create an excitement somewhat akin to what Howard Carter felt in 1922 when he first opened the sealed door to the tomb of Tutankamen. Here is a vast collection of materials, until now largely hidden, which cast a new kind of light on certain aspects of the civilization from which they come. In addition to what is immediately perceived by the observer—scholar, historian, humanist, or interested layman—the materials here represent a rich resource for further study, just as King Tut's artifacts have kept scholars and writers busy for more than half a century.

Indeed, to carry the analogy a bit further, one can say that what we are privileged to find in this book is not so much like the jumbled assortment that Carter found and laboriously sorted and identified, as it is like the amazing King Tut exhibit that toured the United States in the late seventies. The pieces in that collection had the advantage of the best in modern archaeological analysis and identification and the best of modern museumship in their orderly display. Their presentation enhanced the understanding of their historical significance as well as the aesthetic experience of the beholder. A visitor who viewed the same items as they were displayed in the Cairo Museum could well appreciate what the curators of the traveling exhibit had accomplished. The basic materials, by their selection, multifaceted arrangement, occasional restoration, and lighting, became more intelligible and more challenging, raising with great cogency the question: "What do they mean?"

So, David Braddock has likewise delved into dusty archives, assembled and sorted data and supporting interpretive information, and has presented his material with all of the enhancement that modern computer technology makes possible. Prolific computer graphics give immediacy to the tabular presentations in a manner possible only because of the ease and economy with which they can now be produced. From his massive spreadsheet, Braddock has been able to generate matrices and correlations that make many trends of the last half-century instantly observable. Thus, he has made available to the next generation of scholars, policy analysts, and activists not merely raw data, but data organized and sourced, ready for the many off-computer studies and other uses that it can engender and facilitate.

While Braddock's hallmark has been his capacity to apply the highest computer technology to enormous quantities of MR/DD data, with useful results, in this book he has gone further: he has annotated his chapters with legislative and other historical material that not only makes the rise and fall and the redisposition of programs more intelligible, but also supplies important reference points by which one who is interested in social trends may be able to link changes in the status of individual programs (as well as their aggregates) to changes in the social and political climate.

To assist the reader to relate these data to fluctuations in economic conditions, Braddock has supplied here, as he has in earlier publications, detailed comparisons over time in both actual and constant (real) dollars. This volume does not, however, incorporate comparisons with gross national product or aggregate personal income, except in the final chapter. For more detailed analyses, we must look to another major work (Braddock, Hemp, & Howes, 1984). Braddock also gives us some global comparisons between MR/DD expenditures and "the domestic budgetary sector." Clearly, MR/DD rode a rising tide, but gained even by comparison in the period from 1935 to about 1980. Now its decline may also be more pronounced.

The overall upward trend has had its fast and slow periods. An important component in fluctuations can be found in delayed response time. At least three factors contribute to lags between the time a policy change is undertaken and the time that its effects become manifest. Two are obvious—the deliberations of the legislative process itself, particularly at the federal level, and the start-up time needed to move into high gear after legislation is enacted. This delay is usually measured in years, and is further prolonged when the federal policy has to be effectuated through agencies in the respective states. For example, although the legislation authorizing the inclusion of intermediate care services for mentally retarded persons was signed in January, 1972, the final regulations were not published until 1974 and it was 1981 before the present utilizers (every state except Arizona and Wyoming, plus the District of Columbia) had all come on board.

A third factor, often not sufficiently appreciated, is the "real time" phenomenon. There is still a delay in "feedback." We have learned that space flight is greatly facilitated by the capacity of modern computers to "crunch" data as the conditions that generate it are occurring, thus making possible almost instantaneous course corrections. Such analysis is also already applicable to the stock market, but this technology is only beginning to become applicable to the study of social trends. In the absence of reliable telemetry, it will be important to verify the connections between any particular legislation or other stimulating event on the one hand, and bend points in Braddock's data on the other. Moreover, we (like the archaeologists) frequently still find it necessary to interpolate or extrapolate, and for some of his series Braddock has had to do just that, particularly where he has attempted to disaggregate data applicable to MR or DD populations from data tabulated under other rubrics. The reader/researcher is cautioned to read Braddock's careful qualifying notes. The critical instabilities now apparent in our federal spending patterns call on us to be particularly cautious about linear extrapolations and to look for higher order indices. These may be implicit in many but not all of Braddock's data.

Our less than instantaneous ability to identify second order changes (that is, changes in the rate of change) in social and economic indicia in the past has often led to closing the barn door after the horse has fled, simply because we could not track the movements of the horse in timely fashion. For example, in 1980, Congress passed legislation to curtail the number of people and the size of individual benefits awarded under the disability provisions of the Social Security Act. The momentum for this legislation came from an observation that the number of awards in the early seventies was increasing faster than anticipated. By the time the legislation became law, however, it was already apparent that the phenomenon was a temporary one and had begun to subside by 1977. As a result, the 1980 amendments generated overkill, the full impact of which was felt most strongly by disabled Social Security beneficiaries in 1982.

The delay in compiling and analyzing time-series data of this sort has recently been substantially shortened by current computer technology. At the time this book was assembled in 1985, it included verifiable data for 1984 and, in some instances, sound estimates for 1985, a situation never attained for federal statistics in prior decades. This gives a new dimension to the potentials for increasing human productivity. In this book, there is food for much creative research and for thoughtful policy analysis requiring the application of human intelligence. Let us hope it will happen very soon.

Elizabeth M. Boggs, Ph.D.

Acknowledgments

I AM GRATEFUL to all of the individuals in federal government agencies who responded to my numerous and often complex requests for data and interpretive assistance on the operation of their programs. These individuals are listed by name in the references section of the book beginning on page 193. I wish to specifically acknowledge the diligent assistance of Ruth Howes in the collection of data. Leslie Chapital prepared drafts of the original manuscript and along with Richard Hemp tirelessly helped proofread them. Larry Prebis and Steve Garcia generated the book's extensive graphics. Susan Hughes Gray handled the technical editing at Brookes Publishing with efficiency and grace.

I would be remiss in this acknowledgment not to thank two persons who encouraged me and helped to shape my understanding of federal policy in the mental retardation and developmental disabilities field. They are Wallace K. Babington, former executive director of the U.S. Department of Health, Education, and Welfare's Secretary's Committee on Mental Retardation, and the late Professor Jasper Harvey, former chairman of the Department of Special Education at the University of Texas at Austin.

Anyone who writes about the historical aspects of the subject addressed in this book comes to appreciate more acutely the great contributions of Elizabeth Boggs and Gunnar Dybwad. I have merely written about an era they have fundamentally influenced and I am personally grateful for the preface and epilogue they contributed, and for their friendship over the years.

Much of the research on this book was actually carried out 14 years ago and culminated in my doctoral dissertation at the University of Texas at Austin. The present volume can be seen as proof of the academic adage that one never really completes one's dissertation but rather refines and updates it. I would like to acknowledge the original members of that dissertation committee: the late Professor Jasper Harvey; and Professors Laurence Haskew, John D. King (Chair), John R. Peck, and William G. Wolfe.

Finally, I acknowledge the assistance of both the Administration on Developmental Disabilities in the U.S. Department of Health and Human Services and the National Institute of Handicapped Research in the U.S. Department of Education. These two agencies are jointly supporting our ongoing research on the economics of disability. I am also especially grateful to Jean K. Elder, Assistant Secretary of Human Development Services, for her interest and support.

Federal Policy
toward
Mental Retardation
and
Developmental Disabilities

Introduction to the Study

THIS BOOK IS both an analysis of contemporary federal policies in mental retardation and an archival reference document. It was developed for policymakers, professionals, interested laypersons, and students who seek a deeper understanding of the federal role in providing services, personnel training, research, income maintenance, and the construction of facilities for persons with mental retardation or closely related developmental disabilities.

Governmental programs are rooted in the past. Federal programs are rarely created totally anew, but rather are usually grafted to existing statutory and administrative structures. To understand current federal policy in mental retardation/developmental disabilities (MR/DD), one must be familiar with the historical record of myriad individual federal MR/DD program elements, and one must also appreciate each individual element's relation to its broader programmatic environment, its fiscal context, and its legislative history. The prime rationale for this book was the absence of any single document providing this contextual information that also critically analyzed trends in federal policy over time.

The first two chapters, which constitute Part I of the book, provide a nontechnical overview of the history of federal aid in the MR/DD field. Chapters 3–8 (Part II) present in-depth profiles of each individual MR/DD program element supported by the federal government since 1935. There are 82 such profiles, each containing comprehensive information on the element's statutory history, financial record, and programmatic accomplishments.

Chapter 3 addresses federally supported services programs, Chapter 4—personnel training, Chapter 5—research, Chapter 6—income maintenance, Chapter 7—construction, and Chapter 8—information-coordination activities. The financial and programmatic data presented in Chapters 3–8 form the basis of the comprehensive analysis and summary of trends in federal MR/DD policy that appear in Chapter 9. The book concludes with an epilogue by Gunnar Dybwad, professor emeritus of human development at Brandeis University. A reference section that features bibliographical citations and key federal and nonfederal agency respondents follows.

This book presents the results of the federal analysis component of the MR/DD Expenditure Analysis Project. The overall study had three components: the State Government Expenditure Analysis (Braddock, 1986d; Braddock & Fujiura, in press; Braddock, Hemp, & Howes, 1984, 1986); the Analysis of Federal Expenditures (presented herein); and the Intergovernmental Analysis (Braddock & Hemp, 1986). The State Government Expenditure Analysis identified and described state government spending patterns for financing community and institutional services in the United States. It covered the FY 1977–84 period and dealt primarily with state general fund expenditures of the principal MR/DD state agency; the state's utilization of federal ICF/MR (intermediate care facilities for the mentally retarded) reimbursements, and its utilization of the Title XX Social Services Block Grant. The state-focused analysis extended to each of the 50 states and the District of Columbia.

The primary purpose of the State Government Expenditure Analysis was to improve professionals' and policymakers' understanding of important fiscal and programmatic trends that have taken place in many states and at the federal level in recent years. In the

1970s, for example, Nebraska, Minnesota, and many other states implemented major new priorities in financing MR/DD services. These new policies involved more extensive use of state and federal funds for supporting community-based services as alternatives to institutional care. A comprehensive analysis of public MR/DD expenditures on a state-by-state basis would thus reveal the extent to and manner in which states leading the community care movement were financially underwriting community services development. It would also identify those states which, for whatever reasons, were lagging behind the national leaders in this area. The implicit assumption was that an MR/DD service system dominated by community alternatives could not exist without dominant community services funding. (For an extended discussion of the economics of community-based developmental services, see Castellani [in press].)

The second component of the study—the Analysis of Federal Government Expenditures herein reported—had a rationale and research design distinct from, but complementary to, the state government study. The U.S. government provides a good deal more federal resources for the support of MR/DD activities than was reflected in the narrow federal design of the State Government Expenditure Analysis, which considered specifically only Title XIX ICF/MR reimbursements under Medicaid and Title XX/Social Services Block Grant funding. The federal analysis, therefore, was designed to be programmatically comprehensive in scope, analyzing data from all 82 federal MR/DD programs in the areas of services, personnel training, research, income maintenance, construction, and information and coordination. The federal analysis was also historically comprehensive, encompassing the FY 1935–85 period, and not merely FY 1977–84, as was the case with the state government component of the study.

The third component of the study was an Intergovernmental Analysis that integrated the unduplicated financial data emanating from the state and the federal government expenditure studies into a single, unified intergovern-

mental analysis. State and local funds not previously included in the state or federal analyses were infused into the analytical model at this stage. These funds included state and local special education funds, and local government noneducational expenditures for MR/DD services.

The role of expenditure studies in the broader field of policy analysis begins with the explicit conceptual linkage between the expenditures and public policy in the given area of expenditure. The theoretical framework underlying expenditure studies is the classic concept of a responding political system described by Easton (1965). The political system consists of three interrelated parts: 1) political inputs such as citizen needs mediated through the organized demand structure of political parties and special interests; 2) decision-making agencies (executive and legislative agencies, and the judiciary); and 3) policy outputs, including statutes, expenditures, executive orders, and judicial decrees. An expenditure study "measures" the relative scope and intensity of political system outputs—using funds budgeted as the indicator of policy-in-action in the particular area of interest.

Studies of government policy-making have frequently relied solely on revenue and spending data to measure policy. Hofferbert (1972), in his extensive review of state and local policy studies, termed such measures "intermediate output indicators." The budgeting of funds is often the most convenient fiscal record available in the administrative files of executive agencies and legislative bodies. Because the information is quantified, there is also a certain attraction to both the statistical possibilities and to the subtle impression of precision yielded from working with numbers. "From the standpoint of ease and rigor of analysis," Hofferbert has observed, "the advantages of relying on spending and revenue figures are obvious" (1972, p. 36).

Wildavsky (1975) has advocated the use of budgetary data in policy studies because they are readily quantifiable and less warped by subjective judgment than most other analytical indicators. When budgets are studied, one works implicitly with a politics of choice. Because government resources are limited, allocative constraints are always imposed upon the participants. Constituencies such as those interested in MR/DD policy actions are literally told how well their interests are faring in the state house and in Washington by written and verbal reports of dollar distributions. In turn, these constituencies direct political influence in accord with what those reports show or fail to show.

The indicators chosen to represent policy should be understood by the affected consumer population or their advocates, and by key policymakers as relating to the underlying concepts being studied. Johnson (1975) has argued that for policy research "the ultimate test of the validity of indicators as well as the value of our research therefore must be external to our research community" (p. 89). "Every set of measures is a partial representation—is in fact, a kind of mini-theory which hypothesizes the relation between concepts and indicators" (Johnson, 1975, p. 83). Heal and Fujiura (1984) termed this notion of relating indicators to the consumer population "social validity."

The theory implicit in this book is that the care of persons with mental retardation or closely related developmental disabilities in community settings is an ascendant political value across the nation generally, and in most individual states. The care of persons with mental retardation or developmental disabilities in institutional settings is at best only a stable political value, and it is a descendant one in many states. Testing these assumptions using state-federal expenditures over time to index the political values assigned to MR/DD institutional and community services was a major feature of the investigation.

Spending figures in isolation, however, tell one little or nothing about the quality of programs, the fairness with which funds are deployed, nor the relative efficiency with which these dollars are spent. Thus, generalization solely from a fiscal perspective for any complex human services area like mental disability is, although useful and important, lim-ited. Analysis must go beyond mere budget figures and make operational other meaningful indicators of public policy-in-action (Gray, 1980; Johnson, 1975; Rose, 1973). In this particular study, a great deal of programmatic data on the 82 federal program elements was gathered from federal archives, agency records, personal interviews, and government publications.

PURPOSE OF THE ANALYSIS OF FEDERAL POLICY

Presidential committees (President's Panel on Mental Retardation [President's Panel], 1962; President's Task Force on the Mentally Handicapped [President's Task Force], 1970; White House Conference on Handicapped Individuals [White House Conference], 1980), independent study groups (American Bar Association [ABA], 1978), and individual investigators (Braddock, 1973, 1974, 1981; Caiden, 1976; Conley & Noble, 1985; Stedman, Richmond, & Tarjan, 1984; Wieck & Bruininks, 1980) have frequently recommended the systematic collection and analysis of comprehensive financial and programmatic data on the federal government's mental retardation and developmental disabilities programs. The need for such data for planning and program development has been particularly acute since 1974, the year in which the Secretary's Committee on Mental Retardation of the Department of Health, Education, and Welfare (DHEW) was abolished. That coordinating unit, established in 1962, had exercised responsibility for gathering and disseminating technical information on the operation of mental retardation programs within the U.S. Department of Health, Education, and Welfare (Secretary's Committee on Mental Retardation [Secretary's Committee], 1963). Also, since 1974, the federal role in mental retardation has been dramatically expanded with the implementation of many new and large programs such as ICF/MR, Supplemental Security Income, and PL 94-142 (the Education for All Handicapped Children Act).

In addition to comprehensively explicating

the growing federal role in mental retardation, a second and equally important purpose of the study was to assess the fiscal impact of the Omnibus Budget Reconciliation Act of 1981 (PL 97-35) on the rate of growth in federal MR/DD spending during FY 1981–85. In 1981, it was widely believed that PL 97-35 and its associated block grants would lead to a diminution in federal funds budgeted for MR/DD programs (Braddock, 1981; Consortium for Citizens with Developmental Disabilities [Consortium], 1984; Gettings, 1981), and in domestic programs, generally (Nathan & Doolittle, 1984). Testing this thesis with specific respect to MR/DD expenditures was a major feature of the investigation. The study was also expected to provide objective federal financial data to enlighten the continuing national debate on controversial resource allocation proposals such as the Community and Family Living Amendments (i.e., H.R.2902 and S.873).

STRUCTURE OF THE ANALYSIS

Collection of federal financial and programmatic data initially involved identifying relevant federal programs for which appropriations had been made and obligations incurred. Relevant programs were identified by examining the body of law authorizing federal domestic programs. Twenty-five statutes were identified as potentially authorizing appropriations for relevant mental retardation and developmental disabilities activities. These enactments were:

1. Agricultural Trade Development Act as Amended
2. Cooperative Research Act as Amended
3. Developmental Disabilities Services & Facilities Construction Act
4. Domestic Volunteer Service Act as Amended
5. Economic Opportunity Act as Amended
6. Education Professions Development Act
7. Elementary and Secondary Education Act as Amended, including the Education of the Handicapped Act

8. Food Stamp Aid Act as Amended
9. Hospital Survey and Construction Act as Amended
10. Impact Aid to Federally Affected Areas
11. Lead Based Paint Poisoning Prevention Act
12. Library Services and Construction Act as Amended
13. Manpower Training Act as Amended
14. Mental Retardation Facilities & Community Mental Health Centers Construction Act as Amended
15. Military Medical Benefits Act as Amended
16. National Defense Education Act as Amended
17. National Housing Act as Amended
18. National Industrial Recovery Act
19. Omnibus Budget Reconciliation Act of 1981
20. Public Health Services Act as Amended
21. Small Business Act as Amended
22. Social Security Act as Amended
23. Surplus Property Act of 1944 as Amended
24. Vocational Education Act as Amended
25. Vocational Rehabilitation Act as Amended

The 25 statutes contained numerous titles, sections, and subsections authorizing relevant mental retardation and developmental disabilities activities. An MR/DD program element was defined as a specific activity authorized by one of these statutes—or by administrative directive—supporting the provision of services, training of personnel, conduct of research, payments of income maintenance, construction of facilities, or the dissemination of information. A program element was considered relevant to MR/DD only after a review of federal program statistics and administrative records indicated that it provided discrete support for activities benefiting persons with mental retardation or closely related developmental disabilities such as cerebral palsy, epilepsy, or autism. The term "developmental disability" and the acronym "MR/DD" are used in this book to refer to a condition characterized by the presence of mental retardation in either a primary or secondary diagnosis. (When mental retardation is present as a secondary diagnosis, for example, the primary diagnosis is frequently cerebral palsy.)

It must also be made clear that the term developmental disability first appeared in federal statute in 1970 in PL 91-517. Hence, programmatic references in the book predating 1970 will usually refer strictly to "mentally retarded" recipients of service. Generally, however, the reader may infer that recipients with developmental disabilities closely related to mental retardation were also served in "mental retardation" programs. In total, 82 MR/DD program elements were

identified during the course of the study. These are presented in Table 1.

To facilitate replication of the study, sources of all data, including any cost-analysis techniques employed, are described in detail in Part II of this volume. The primary source of MR/DD financial data was the administrative records of agency financial management units and program offices. Congressional memoranda transmitting appropriation bills, budget justifications, records of congressional appropriation hearings, the annual budget of the federal government, and Department of Health and Human Services archives were also important data sources.

An analytical profile of each of the 82 MR/DD program elements presenting each el-

Table 1. Federal program elements supporting MR/DD expenditures since 1935

I. SERVICES
  A. Educational Services
    1. Special Education (ESEA)
      1.1 Title I, PL 89-313: Aid to State Schools
      1.2 Title II, Elementary and Secondary Education Act: Aid to State School Libraries
      1.3 Title VI B 94-142: State Grants
      1.4 Title VI B, PL 94-142: Preschool Incentive Grants
      1.5 Title VI C, Sec. 621: Regional Resource Centers
      1.6 Title VI C, Sec. 623: Early Childhood Projects
      1.7 Title VI C, Sec. 624: Severely Handicapped Projects
      1.8 Title VI C, Sec. 622: Centers for Deaf-Blind Children
      1.9 Title VI F, Instructional Media
    2. Vocational Education
      2.1 PL 90-576 as Amended: State Grants
    3. Impact Aid
      3.1–3.3 PL 81-874, Sec. 3(a) and (b) Special Education, Indian Special Education
  B. Vocational Rehabilitation Services
    1. Title I, PL 93-112 as Amended: State Grants
    2. Sec. 13, Vocational Rehabilitation Act: Facility Improvement Grants
    3. Sec. 3, Vocational Rehabilitation Act: Extension & Improvement Grants
  C. Public Health Services
    1. DHHS-Public Health Service
      1.1 Title XIX, Social Security Act: ICF/MR Program
      1.2 Title XIX, Social Security Act: Non-Institutional Medicaid
      1.3 Title XVIII, Social Security Act: Medicare
      1.4 Title V, Sec. 503, Maternal & Child Health Grants
      1.5 Title V, Sec. 504, Crippled Children's Grants
      1.6 Sec. 314 (c & e), Public Health Services Act
      1.7 PL 91-695: Lead Based Paint Poisoning Prevention
      1.8 PL 88-156: State Planning in Mental Retardation
    2. Dept. of Defense - CHAMPUS
  D. Human Development Services
    1. Developmental Disabilities Act (HDS)
      1.1 Part B, PL 88-164 as Amended: UAF Grants
      1.2 Part C, PL 88-164 as Amended: State Grants
      1.3 Part D, PL 88-164 as Amended: Staffing Grants
      1.4 Sec. 145 D, PL 88-164 as Amended: Special Projects
      1.5 Sec. 113, PL 88-164 as Amended: P & A Grants
    2. Other HDS Administered Services
      2.1 Title XX, Social Services Block Grant, Social Security Act as Amended, 1962
      2.2 Social Security Act as Amended, Child Welfare Services

(continued)

Table 1. (*continued*)

2.3 Economic Opportunity Act of 1964 as Amended (Head Start)
3. Action Agency
   3.1 Domestic Volunteer Service Act of 1973
4. Department of Labor
   4.1 Job Training Partnership Act of 1962 as Amended

II. TRAINING OF PERSONNEL

A. Training of Special Education Personnel
   1. PL 88-164 as Amended
   2. PL 90-35, Education Professions Development Act
B. Training of Rehabilitation Personnel
   1. Vocational Rehabilitation Act of 1954 as Amended
C. Training of Health Services Personnel
   1. National Institutes of Health
      1.1 PL 87-838, Sec. 411, Public Health Services Act Title IV E (NICHD)
      1.2 Public Health Services Act, Title IV D (NINCDS)
   2. Maternal & Child Health Services Training
      2.1 Social Security Act, Title V, Sec. 511, Mothers & Children
      2.2 Social Security Act, Title V, Sec. 503, Maternal & Child Health
      2.3 Social. Security Act, Title V, Sec. 504, Crippled Children
   3. Public Health Services Act, Sec. 303

III. RESEARCH

A. Educational Research
   1. Title VI E, PL 91-230 (EHA): Special Education Research
   2. Title III, Supplementary Services
   3. Title IV, Innovation and Support
   4. National Defense Education Act of 1958: Media Research
   5. PL 83-531: Cooperative Research Act
B. Rehabilitation Research & Demonstration
   1. VR Research—NIHR
      1.1 Mental Retardation Research & Training
      1.2 Other Research-Sec. 204(a)(2)(A)/202(a)
      1.3 Other Research-Sec.4(a)(1)
      1.4 PL 83-480: Foreign Currency Research
   2. Special Demonstrations
      2.1 Sec. 311, Rehabilitation Act of 1973 as Amended: Severely Disabled Demonstrations
      2.2 Sec. 621, Rehabilitation Act of 1973 as Amended: Projects with Industry
      2.3 Sec. 316, Vocational Rehabilitation Act of 1978 as Amended:

Special Recreation Demonstrations
C. Biomedical & Health Services Research
   1. Nat. Inst. of Health: Biomedical Research
      1.1 PL 87-838, Title IV E, Sec. 411—NICHD
      1.2 PL 87-838, Title IV D—NINCDS
      1.3 PL 81-962, Title IV, Public Health Services Act of 1950 as Amended: NIAID
   2. Other Health Research: NIMH/MCH
      2.1 Mental Health Research, NIMH, Public Health Services Act, Sec. 301
      2.2 Sec. 303, Public Health Services Act: Hospital Improvement Projects
      2.3 Health Services Research, Social Security Act, Title V, Sec. 512

IV. INCOME MAINTENANCE

A. Appropriated Funds
   1. Aid to the Permanently & Totally Disabled: Social Security Act, Title XIV
   2. Supplemental Security Income: Social Security Act, Title XVI
   3. Food Stamp Aid: PL 95-113
   4. Supplemental Security Income: Social Security Act, Title XVI, Sec. 1615
B. Trust Funds
   1. Adult Disabled Child: Social Security Act, Title II, Sec. 202(a)
   2. Title II, Sec. 222

V. CONSTRUCTION

A. NIRA of 1933: Grants & Loans (Total NIRA)
   1. NIRA of 1933 Grants
   2. NIRA of 1933 Loans
B. Surplus Property Act of 1944, as Amended (DHHS)
C. Health Facilities: Hill-Burton Act
D. PL 88-164: Mental Retardation Facilities Grants
   1. Part A—Research Centers
   2. Part B—UAF Construction
   3. Part C—Community Facilities
E. PL 91-517—Developmental Disabilities Formula Grants Construction
F. Rehabilitation Facility Construction Grants (Sec. 12)
G. Housing Loans: HUD Act, Sec. 202
H. Small Business Act of 1953, as Amended

VI. INFORMATION & COORDINATION

A. President's Panel on Mental Retardation
B. Secretary's Committee on Mental Retardation
C. President's Committee on Mental Retardation

ement's statutory purpose and legislative history is presented in Part II of this book (Chapters 3–8). Part II is intended to be used as an archival reference rather than as a continuous analytical narrative. The profiles include computer-generated graphics depicting the programmatic and financial history of each of the individual program elements. When available, performance data were included on clients served, projects funded, clinics opened, etc. Part III of this volume (Chapter 9) presents an analytical overview and summary of the entire study.

The analysis of federal data presented in Chapters 3–8 is classified into six activity categories, as shown in Table 1: services, training of personnel, research, income maintenance, construction, and information and coordination. (The profiles of the 82 MR/DD program elements in Chapters 3–8 are presented sequentially in these 6 activity categories.) Data are subclassified into program areas by discipline (i.e., public health, special education, rehabilitation, and human development services). Income maintenance program elements are classified into appropriated and trust funds.

For analytical convenience, all financial data were organized chronologically into an electronic spreadsheet using a microcomputer equipped with a digital plotting device. The spreadsheet yielded annual totals for FY 1935–85 for the 82 program elements and each activity category, and also by administering agency. Data were also analyzed both in unadjusted and real economic terms (constant dollars) using the state and local subindex of the Gross National Product (GNP) implicit price deflator (Bureau of Economic Analysis, 1984). An analysis of trends was completed for year-to-year expenditures in each activity category, by agency, and for each individual program element. Two economic scales were used to measure the relative growth or "fiscal effort" reflected in federal MR/DD spending over time: percentage of the GNP; and percentage of the federal government's total annual budget. Fiscal effort is discussed in Chapter 9.

In the following two chapters, the history of federal assistance for MR/DD activities is described. This is primarily a legislative history providing certain background technical information necessary to a fuller understanding of subsequent chapters in this volume and of the contemporary federal MR/DD mission in general.

PART I

FEDERAL ASSISTANCE FOR MENTAL RETARDATION AND DEVELOPMENTAL DISABILITIES

Chapter 1

Federal Assistance
for Mental Retardation
and Developmental Disabilities
through 1961

FEDERAL GOVERNMENT PROGRAMS concerned with mental retardation and developmental disabilities have grown rapidly in recent decades. Programs adopted have ranged from support of basic scientific research at the National Institutes of Health to federal reimbursements of expenditures for habilitative services in state-operated institutions. The adoption of 82 federal mental retardation and developmental disabilities program elements during FY 1935–85 is depicted in Figure 1. No more than 56 program elements were operational in any single year. Figure 1 presents cumulative operational elements on an annual basis.

The purpose of this chapter is to describe the evolution of federal government mental retardation assistance programs prior to the issuance of President John F. Kennedy's October 11, 1961, "Statement on the Need for a National Plan in Mental Retardation" (President's Panel on Mental Retardation [President's Panel],1962).

Chapter 2 addresses the modern era of 1962–85. Unless otherwise noted, the source of all financial data and legislative material is delineated in Chapters 3–8 of this volume. Previous work by Boggs (1971; 1972), Brad-

dock (1973; 1974), and by the Office for Handicapped Individuals (OHI; 1980) was especially helpful in the preparation of this chapter and of Chapter 2. Both chapters, however, were primarily developed using primary data sources such as archives and administrative records of federal agencies and the United States Congress.

FORMATIVE DEVELOPMENTS: GRANTS-IN-AID

Public Health

In 1798, the Fifth Congress passed the first federal law concerned with the care of persons with disabilities. It authorized a Marine Hospital Service financed by levies collected by customs agents in United States ports. The levies were deducted from the wages of merchant seamen, and only sick or disabled seamen were eligible to receive care. Around 1900, the service became responsible for the control of cummunicable diseases when the states, according to Mountin, "either failed or refused to enforce program quarantine measures" (1949, p. 83). The service's name was also changed to the Public Health and Marine

An adaptation of this chapter appeared in: Braddock, D. (1986a). Federal assistance for mental retardation and developmental disabilities: A review through 1961. *Mental Retardation, 24* (3), 175–182.

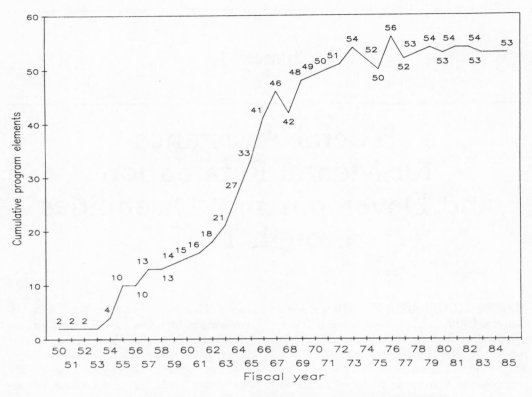

Figure 1.   The adoption of federal MR/DD program elements over time: FY 1950–85.

Hospital Service to reflect its expanded responsibilities.

In 1912, the name was simplified to its contemporary designation—the U.S. Public Health Service (PHS). Four years later, $25,000 was appropriated to the PHS for studies and demonstrations in rural sanitation. Federal funds had to be matched on a one-to-one basis with state monies. In 1921, the nation's first health services formula grant program was authorized: the Maternity and Infancy Act, or Sheppard-Towner. The act operated for 8 years and expired in 1929. Sheppard-Towner was the predecessor of Title V (Sections 503 and 504) of the Social Security Act of 1935, which authorized state formula grants for Maternal and Child Health and Crippled Children's Services.

Vocational Education and Rehabilitation

The years 1917–21 were formative for federal grant programs in education and vocational rehabilitation. The Smith-Hughes Act of 1917 authorized grants to states for vocational education activities. This program was not only the first major federal program in public education; it was the nation's first state formula grant program in the broad health/education/welfare arena. However, services to persons with disabilities were not authorized.

The nation's oldest federal program authorizing services to civilians with disabilities was enacted in 1920, as the Smith-Fess Act, otherwise known as the Civilian Vocational Rehabilitation Act of 1920 (OHI, 1980). Two years earlier, PL 65–178 had authorized rehabilitation services to discharged military personnel with physical disabilities (LaVor, 1975). The Smith-Fess Act established a reimbursement program requiring a dollar-for-dollar state match, although no services were provided to individuals with mental disabilities. In 1935, the act was incorporated into

Title V of the landmark Social Security Act. That legislation doubled the previous authorization level for rehabilitation reimbursements, to $2 million annually. In 1939, the authorization level was increased to $3.5 million per year.

Children's Bureau Studies

Excluding the activities of the U.S. Census Bureau, which began enumerating persons with mental retardation in the 1840 decennial census (Boggs, 1971), the first discrete federal mental retardation activity was the commissioning of three epidemiological and sociological studies by the U.S. Children's Bureau. These studies of "mental defect" were published by the bureau as a part of its "Dependent, Defective, and Delinquent Classes Publication Series" in 1915 (U.S. Children's Bureau), 1917 (Lundberg), and 1919 (Treadway & Lundberg).

The investigators examined the status of and documented the need for services to persons with mental retardation in the District of Columbia; New Castle County, Delaware; and Sussex County, Delaware, respectively. The bureau published dozens of similar pathbreaking studies on such subjects as infant mortality, child labor, and child welfare. It was nearly 2 decades later, however, before the bureau was vested with grant-in-aid authority under the Social Security Act to begin addressing the nationwide problems it had so ably identified.

THE GREAT DEPRESSION AND SOCIAL SECURITY

Public Works Administration

The Great Depression presented Washington with nationwide problems that, many Americans widely believed, only a nationwide government could resolve. In President Franklin Roosevelt's first term, Congress enacted the National Industrial Recovery Act of 1933 (NIRA). This legislation established the Public Works Administration which, during FY 1933–39, processed $5.49 billion in federal

construction grants and loans (Short & Stanley-Brown, 1939). By 1938, 27,650 buildings had been erected with federal assistance throughout the United States.

Short and Stanley-Brown (1939) described a sample of 620 architecturally representative projects, or about 8% of all those funded by NIRA through FY 1937. Inspection of these project descriptions revealed that about $16.5 million was budgeted during FY 1935–39 by the federal government for construction projects located at 14 state psychiatric hospitals and 2 mental retardation institutions. Total federal construction expenditures at mental institutions could have been as high as $200 million during the Depression, assuming the Short and Stanley-Brown sample was representative. Moreover, 10%–15% of the residents of state mental hospitals during this period were individuals with a primary diagnosis of mental retardation (Office of Mental Retardation Coordination [OMRC], 1972).

Social Security Act of 1935

The Social Security Act of 1935 did not originally authorize public assistance for persons with disabilities, other than a small Aid to the Blind Program authorized by Title X. The original act also authorized Old Age Assistance (Title I), and Aid to Families with Dependent Children (Title IV). Persons with mental disabilities, however, relied only on "General Assistance," which was financed by more than 10,000 local administrative units, some with state assistance. Local assistance agencies could not use federal funds under Titles I, IV, or X to supply medical care; and few state agencies authorized this type of expenditure. Falk and Geddes (1941) observed that "the burden of medical care, in so far as it is borne by public authorities, falls upon General [relief] agencies" (p. 68).

A decade after the enactment of Social Security legislation, America's 19 largest cities budgeted nearly 50% of all funds expended in this country for General Assistance, even though those cities constituted only 20% of the total United States general population. A report prepared in 1946 for the U.S. House of

Representatives Ways and Means Committee described General Assistance as "extremely meager in some counties and in others totally lacking" (U.S. House of Representatives [House], 1946, p. 301).

Maternal and Child Health and Crippled Children's Services

Title VI of the Social Security Act authorized appropriations of $8 million annually for grants to states to establish and maintain state and local public health authorities. Title V of the act also authorized grants to states for Maternal and Child Health and Crippled Children's Services. Totals of $3.8 million and $2.85 million, respectively, were authorized for the two programs. Both of these programs, however, had not been designed to deal with the problems of children with mental handicaps. The minutes of the 1936 board meeting of the Crippled Children's Services National Advisory Committee contained the recommendation that "children with incurable blindness, deafness, or mental defect . . . and those requiring permanent custodial care should be beyond the scope of the Program" (Social Security Board, 1946, p. 1).

A decade later, however, the same committee met jointly with its counterpart in the Maternal and Child Health Program and called attention to the large number of children with "cerebral palsy . . . and epilepsy" (Social Security Board, 1946, p. 5). A joint recommendation was issued to conduct a fact-finding survey of the incidence and prevalence of cerebral palsy. Medical school training programs in this area were also encouraged. The committees also called for the Children's Bureau to hire a full-time mental health specialist and encouraged federal, state, and local agencies to establish child guidance clinics with broadly construed mental hygiene functions. Although amendments to Title V increased the program's authorization levels in 1939 and 1946, federally supported Maternal and Child Health and Crippled Children's Services to children with developmental disabilities were extremely limited until the late 1950s.

WORLD WAR II AND ITS AFTERMATH

Barden-LaFollete

During the 1939–45 period, the federal government was preoccupied with waging a worldwide war. State governments felt the economic shock—public expenditures for state institutions actually fell in real economic terms during the war (Lakin, 1979). With one important exception, there was virtually no federal legislative progress in the MR/DD field. In 1943, Congress enacted the Barden-LaFollete Act, which amended vocational rehabilitation legislation with provisions authorizing services to mentally handicapped individuals. In 1945, the first year the amendment was implemented, 106 persons nationwide who were mentally retarded (most of whom lived in Michigan) were reported rehabilitated under the state-federal grant program. This was .3% of the total rehabilitation caseload that year (OMRC, 1972).

The first successful federally funded demonstration efforts in training, counseling, and placement of individuals with mental retardation occurred prior to 1950 (Braddock, 1974). After the Second World War, the number of clients with mental retardation rehabilitated increased steadily. Amendments to the act in 1954 expanded available resources and the caseload. In FY 1955, 531 persons with mental retardation were reported rehabilitated under the state-federal program. This was .9% of the nationwide rehabilitation caseload.

Surplus Property

The Surplus Property Act of 1944 authorized the executive branch to dispose of certain federally owned real and personal properties. Properties available literally ranged from large army hospitals to helicopter seats. Since 1955, the program has been responsible for the transfer of $28 million in land and buildings to MR/DD uses by state, local, and nonprofit service providers. The program was particularly active during, and shortly after, the presidency of John F. Kennedy (Office of Real Property, 1984; U.S. House of Representatives [House], 1963).

Aid to the Permanently and Totally Disabled (APTD)

Under the original Social Security Act, a person with mental retardation could receive state-federal assistance only if he or she qualified for assistance as "old" under the definition set forth in Title I, as a "dependent child" per Title IV, or as a "blind" individual as authorized by Title X. The Social Security Amendments of 1950 changed the original act to authorize a program of "Aid to the Permanently and Totally Disabled" (OHI, 1980). This allowed persons with severe disabilities to qualify for state-federal public assistance. The APTD Program operated for nearly 25 years before it was revised and expanded in 1972 by the Supplemental Security Income (SSI) Program.

Mental Health and Neurological Disorders Research and Training

The National Mental Health Act of 1946 added another key organization to the growing number of federal agencies that would later play a major role in the federal mental retardation effort. Initially, there was little activity in mental retardation at the National Institute of Mental Health (NIMH), which had been created by the act. During the FY 1956 House budget hearings, however, NIMH Director Robert Felix cited discretionary mental retardation research and training support for seven FY 1955 projects totaling $121,064 (Braddock, 1973). Legislation in 1950 amending Title IV of the Public Health Service Act established the National Institute of Neurological Diseases and Blindness (NINDB), now the National Institute of Neurological and Communicative Disorders and Stroke (NINCDS). The institute assumed responsibility for supporting research in cerebral palsy and epilepsy. In 1954, NINDB supported MR/DD research and training projects amounting to $326,000, 7.4% of its total budget (Braddock, 1974).

Diagnostic Clinics

In 1954, the Children's Bureau, originally in the U.S. Department of Labor, was transferred to the Welfare Administration of the newly created Department of Health, Education, and Welfare (DHEW). That year, the bureau provided project grant funds to California for a mental retardation diagnostic clinic. A year later, similar awards were made to Hawaii, the District of Columbia, and the state of Washington for demonstrations of community-based mental retardation clinical services (U.S. Children's Bureau, 1964). Hornmuth (1964) reported that there were no special mental retardation diagnostic clinics in the United States in 1949. About 15 were in operation in 1957. Most clinics were either initiated or being operated by member units of the fledgling National Association for Retarded Children (NARC) (Hornmuth, 1964).

THE FOGARTY COMMITTEE AND DHEW'S RESPONSE

Fogarty's Leadership

In 1955, Congressman John Fogarty, chairman of the Labor-DHEW Appropriations Subcommittee, quizzed testifying DHEW officials including Secretary Ovetta Culp Hobby, about what the department was doing for children with mental retardation. Briefed by NARC supporters, Fogarty came to believe that a great deal could be done to help children who were mentally retarded, and the federal government was not doing its share. In fact, the subcommittee's report on the FY 1958 appropriations bill observed that, "two years ago there was not an identifiable program in the Federal Government aimed at meeting the problem of mentally retarded children" (House, 1963, p. 2).

In 1955, Fogarty's subcommittee earmarked $750,000 in the FY 1956 Labor-DHEW Appropriations Bill for mental retardation research. These funds were appropriated as $500,000 and $250,000 increases over budget requests of the NINDB and the NIMH, respectively. Fogarty's subcommittee also directed the Office of Education to develop a mental retardation program and to present it to the subcommittee one year later (U.S. House of Representatives [House], 1955).

DHEW Committee Appointed

Secretary Hobby returned to DHEW after the February 8, 1955 budget hearings and instructed the staff to form an *ad hoc* internal committee to address the various mental retardation issues Congressman Fogarty had raised. The "Ad Hoc Committee on Mental Retardation on Proposed DHEW Programs, Activities, Services, and Budget Estimates" was thus formed. The committee consisted of 10 representatives from the NINDB, NIMH, Office of Education, Children's Bureau, Office of Vocational Rehabilitation, and the Bureau of Public Assistance in the Social Security Administration. Dr. Joseph Douglass, Assistant to the Assistant Secretary for Legislation in the DHEW, chaired the committee. Fifteen years later he would become the second Executive Director of the President's Committee on Mental Retardation.

The Ad Hoc Committee transmitted its report to Secretary Hobby on May 19, 1955, in an historic 25-page document (U.S. Department of Health, Education, and Welfare [DHEW], 1955). It recommended the secretarial appointment of a standing departmental committee on mental retardation with agency representation similar to the composition of the Ad Hoc Committee, and requested $80,000 for the new committee's operation. The secretary complied with the request. The new committee was the forerunner of the Secretary's Committee on Mental Retardation, established in 1962 to deal with the extra workload imposed on the DHEW by the President's Panel on Mental Retardation. The Ad Hoc Committee's report also recommended a revision of the Hill-Burton Medical Facilities Construction Act to permit the "construction and expansion of public institutions for the feeble-minded" (DHEW, 1955, p. 8); and it presented FY 1957 budget requests in mental retardation for each agency represented on the committee.

The Children's Bureau asked for $77,039 for increased staff salaries and expenses so that consultation with the states on clinical services to infants and preschool retarded children could be expanded. The bureau also recommended increasing the authorization level for Maternal and Child Health Services from $16.5 million to $20 million. The Bureau of Public Assistance indicated that it required $1.5 million for grants to states for research, demonstration, and staff training; and $80,000 for increased staff salaries and expenses. The Office of Education requested $2.073 million, about half of which was earmarked for proposed fellowship support, and the remainder for research on the educational problems of children who were mentally retarded.

Biomedical and Behavioral Research

The NIMH and the NINDB requested $640,000 and $1.265 million, respectively, for extramural and intramural research grants, and for traineeships/fellowships. The NIMH investigations were to be geared to the study of the basic psychological and sociological problems of persons with mental retardation, while NINDB focused its proposed research on studies of genetic, prenatal, perinatal, and other etiological factors.

Rehabilitation Research

The Office of Vocational Rehabilitation (OVR) request was the most detailed and extensive, seeking a total of $2.555 million for FY 1957 activities in mental retardation. Of this sum, $2.5 million was requested for Section 4 (a)(2)(A)—a research program which had only recently been authorized by the Vocational Rehabilitation Act Amendments of 1954. Under its provisions, OVR was empowered to make grants to state agencies or other nonprofit organizations to assist the expansion or initiation of services "holding promise of substantially increasing the number of persons rehabilitated." Inspection of OVR archives revealed 41 mental retardation expansion projects funded by OVR between FY 1955 and 57 (Braddock, 1973).

Summary

In little more than 3 months, the DHEW had responded to Fogarty's stimulus with a total budget request of $7.63 million, excluding the increase in the authorization level requested for State Maternal and Child Health Grants. Over the next 4 years, virtually every recommendation of the Ad Hoc Committee was implemented. For the first time, the federal government had begun to recognize its responsibilities to citizens with mental retardation. Concerned parents provided the impetus for bringing forth this recognition.

PROGRAM EXPANSION: 1956–61

Adult Disabled Child Benefits (ADC)

The congressional legislative agenda for 1956–58 reflected Congressman Fogarty's design for expanded federal mental retardation commitments across the board. The Social Security Act Amendments of 1956 authorized benefits for Adults Disabled in Childhood from Social Security trust funds. Benefits were authorized under Title II, Section 202 (a) to continue after age 18 if the surviving children of retired, deceased, or disabled workers were classified as disabled themselves. During 1957–69, 68% of all ADC recipients were diagnosed as having a mental deficiency. This percentage has fluctuated between 69% and 72% since 1969. Benefit payments to persons with mental retardation were projected to reach $1.273 billion under the ADC Program in FY 1985 (See Chapter 6, Figure 84).

Hospital Construction

Prior to FY 1965, when the Mental Retardation Facilities and Community Mental Health Centers Construction Act was implemented, the Hill-Burton Hospital Construction Program was the primary source of funds for MR/DD facilities construction activity. Sums budgeted ranged from $2.3 million in FY 1960 to $6.5 million in FY 1965. In total, $32 million was expended under the program on 90 mental retardation projects during FY 1958–71. State institutions, workshops, activity centers, and other nonprofit community facilities were assisted under the program (U.S. Department of Health, Education, and Welfare, Health Services and Mental Health Administration, 1972).

Educational Research and Training

Fiscal years 1957–59 were notable for the discretionary grants awarded for research in mental retardation under the Cooperative Research Act (PL 83-531) and the National Defense Education Act (PL 85-864). During this period, obligations under the Cooperative Research Act budgeted for mental retardation research ranged from 65% to 36% of total Cooperative Research Act spending.

Congress also enacted a statute in 1958—PL 85-926—authorizing the first program to train teachers of children with mental retardation. In FY 1960, $985,000 was expended for this purpose in 16 institutions of higher education and in 23 state education agencies. That year, 177 traineeships were sponsored. This act, along with a similar categorical program authorizing the training of teachers of deaf children, was the forerunner of today's special education personnel preparation program in the U.S. Department of Education.

The President's Panel

In 1961, 9 months after John F. Kennedy took the presidential oath of office, he issued a formal statement establishing the President's Panel on Mental Retardation. "We as a nation," he said, "have for too long postponed an intensive search for solutions to the problems of the mentally retarded. That failure should be corrected" (President's Panel, 1962 p. 196). President Kennedy appointed a panel of 27 distinguished physicians, scientists, educators, lawyers, and consumers to chart a "comprehensive and coordinated attack on the problem of mental retardation" (President's Panel, 1962, p. 201). The panel was organized into six task forces: Prevention, Education and Habilitation, Law and Public Resources, Biological Research, Behavioral and Social Research, and Coordination (President's Panel, 1962). The president gave the panel until December 31, 1962 to complete its assignment. In retrospect, the panel symbolized the temporary emergence of the executive branch as the leading political force in the development of the federal government's MR/DD financial assistance programs.

SUMMARY

This chapter has summarized the early historical evolution of federal assistance programs for mental retardation and developmental disabilities in the United States. Assistance programs were traced from the creation of the forerunner of the U.S. Public Health Service in 1798 to the appointment of the President's Panel on Mental Retardation in 1961. Major legislative benchmarks in the early twentieth century were the Vocational Education, Vocational Rehabilitation, and Maternity and Infancy Acts of 1917, 1920, and 1921, respectively; the National Industrial Recovery Act of 1933; and the Social Security Act of 1935, which authorized Maternal and Child Health Services, Crippled Children's Services, Aid to the Blind, and also extended the Vocational Rehabilitation Program.

In 1943, vocational rehabilitation services were extended to individuals with mental disabilities. In 1950, the first federal welfare program for previously nonqualifying persons with severe disabilities was authorized (APTD). Six years later, benefit payments were authorized from Social Security trust funds for adult disabled children of insured workers.

Congress was instrumental in the adoption of five mental retardation assistance programs during FY 1955–61. The U.S. House of Representatives Subcommittee on Labor-DHEW appropriations, chaired by Congressman John Fogarty, stimulated the adoption of assistance programs in research, demonstration of services, and personnel training. As the period drew to a close, President John F. Kennedy issued the first presidential statement on mental retardation and formally established his presidential panel (President's Panel, 1962). With this action, the modern era of federal concern for persons with mental retardation and developmental disabilities began. The history of the modern era is the subject of Chapter 2.

Chapter 2

Federal Assistance
for Mental Retardation
and Developmental Disabilities
in the Modern Era

THE PREVIOUS CHAPTER summarized the evolution of the federal government's mental retardation financial assistance programs through 1961 and the appointment of the President's Panel on Mental Retardation. That historical review is extended in this chapter through the enactment of the Developmental Disabilities Amendments of 1984.

The present chapter addresses what might be termed the modern era of federal assistance. It encompasses the Great Society legislation of the sixties and the Reagan block grants of the eighties. Initiatives are described in social services, public health, special education, developmental disabilities, intermediate care facilities for the mentally retarded (ICFs/MR), Supplemental Security Income (SSI), Adult Disabled Child (ADC) and Social Security benefits, food stamps, housing and business loans, and "Baby Doe." The chapter begins with a discussion of the implementation of the recommendations the President's Panel embodied in PL 88-156 and PL 88-164.

THE PRESIDENT'S PANEL
ON MENTAL RETARDATION

PL 88-156 Enacted

The 95 recommendations of President John F. Kennedy's Panel on Mental Retardation (President's Panel, 1962) form the basis of today's federal assistance programs in the field. The panel's work was broad and far reaching, extending to many facets of scientific inquiry and program development, and to basic issues of justice. Tangible legislative results of the panel's work included the subsequent enactment of PL 88-156—the Maternal and Child Health and Mental Retardation Planning Amendments of 1963. This law doubled authorizations for the Maternal and Child Health State Grant Program and authorized a small 3-year state planning grant program. Part 4 of the act also authorized special Section 508 grants for Maternity and Infant Care, "to help reduce incidence of mental retardation caused by complications associated with childbearing" (Secretary's Com-

An adaptation of this chapter appeared in: Braddock, D. (1986b). Federal assistance for mental retardation and developmental disabilities: The modern era. *Mental Retardation, 24* (4).

mittee on Mental Retardation [Secretary's Committee], 1965).

PL 88-164

PL 88-164, the Mental Retardation Facilities and Community Mental Health Centers Construction Act, became law on October 31, 1963, only a few weeks before the president who had championed its passage was assassinated. The act authorized three interrelated construction programs. Title I, Part A authorized the construction of research centers, and $27 million in Part A funds were expended for the establishment of 12 such centers between FY 1965 and FY 1967. A mental retardation branch at the National Institute of Child Health and Human Development (NICHD) was created to administer the research centers' programs. University Affiliated Facilities (UAFs) were authorized to be built with monies budgeted under Title I, Part B of the act. In total, between FY 1965 and FY 1971, $38.5 million was allocated for UAF construction at 18 sites.

A Community Facilities Construction Program was also authorized under Title I, Part C of the act. This program assisted states in the erection of specially designed facilities for the diagnosis, treatment, education, training, and personal care of people with mental retardation. Of the 3 construction programs sponsored by the act, Part C received the most funds—$90.2 million between FY 1965 and FY 1970 for 362 projects. Part C was to have addressed the need for community services throughout the nation. During FY 1967–68, however, at the height of the Vietnam conflict, funds to implement Part C were presidentially impounded (Braddock, 1973).

Social Services Expanded

The Social Security Act Amendments of 1962 increased the federal matching provision to 75% for Social Services authorized under Titles IV, X, XIV, and XVI. In March, 1962, the Department of Health, Education, and Welfare (DHEW) Secretary issued a new policy directive permitting federal social services

funds to assist persons on conditional release from state mental institutions (U.S. House of Representatives [House], 1963). For the first time, the federal government also agreed, to participate in financing Social Services for recipients of public assistance. This allowed states to significantly broaden services to community residents who were mentally retarded or otherwise developmentally disabled.

The Social Services program grew slowly at first; within a decade its open-end reimbursement feature and favorable match motivated Congress to legislate a $2.5 billion lid on the program. Social Services funds were used in the late sixties in several states, most notably Nebraska, to significantly expand community-based MR/DD services.

DEVELOPMENTS IN SPECIAL EDUCATION: 1963–70

Title III of PL 88-164 was an education bill concealed in health legislation to prevent it from becoming tied up in a civil rights impasse between the Kennedy administration and the Chairman of the House Committee on Education and Labor. The chairman, according to Boggs (1971), had threatened to hold up all education legislation if the administration did not accelerate support for civil rights. To administer Title III, which extended and expanded the teacher training provisions authorized in PL 85-926 and also added a new research authority, a Division on the Education of Handicapped Children was established in the U.S. Office of Education. Its first director, Dr. Samuel Kirk of the University of Illinois, was appointed by President Kennedy in 1963. The new division did not begin actual operation however, until July, 1965 (Martin, 1968).

The Carey Committee

In 1965, New York Congressman Hugh Carey's Ad Hoc House Subcommittee on Handicapped Children held hearings and the result was a substantial expansion of the federal role in special education (U.S. House of Representatives [House], 1966). However, the new Division on the Education of Handicapped Children was dissolved by an agency-wide reorganization in 1966, only one year after its creation. (Implementation of the Elementary and Secondary Education Act of 1965 [ESEA] had, in one year, literally doubled the total appropriation of the U.S. Office of Education.) Congress responded by statutorily mandating, in PL 89-750 (the ESEA Amendments of 1966), the creation of a new Bureau of Education for the Handicapped; it also authorized a State Grant Program under Title VI, Part A, reframed in 1968 as Title VI, Part B. Title VI A was budgeted at only $2.425 million in FY 1967, but the program was greatly expanded 8 years later by the Education for All Handicapped Children Act (PL 94-142).

Education Earmarks

The education agenda was not only expanding in the late sixties through enactments in special education, but also through earmarks applied to "regular" and vocational education. The ESEA Amendments of 1967 stipulated that states had to spend at least 15% of their funds available under the ESEA Title III, a demonstration authority, on projects involving handicapped children. This earmark was retained in legislation enacted 11 years later that reframed Title III as Title IV, Part C of PL 95-561, the ESEA Amendments of 1978.

In 1968, Congress passed PL 90-576, amending the Vocational Education Act to require that 10% of the funds expended under the State Grant Program be allocated for projects serving children with handicaps. Amendments enacted in 1976 extended this provision and also encouraged the integration of handicapped students into regular vocational education programs. In 1972, Congress modified the Economic Opportunity Act (PL 92-424) by requiring that at least 10% of Head Start's enrollment opportunities be reserved for children with handicaps. The authorizing amendments in PL 92-424 defined handicapped children in terms of Section 602 of the Education of the Handicapped Act (EHA, PL 91-230, Title VI).

PL 89-313 and PL 91-230

Soon after the enactment of the original ESEA of 1965 (PL 89-10), advocates discovered that no clear provision had been made to assist handicapped students in state-operated or state-supported schools. The remedy was PL 89-313, an amendment to ESEA, Title I, which extended eligibility for the nation's children and youth residing in state mental retardation institutions and psychiatric hospitals.

The ESEA Amendments of 1970, PL 91-230, established a new Title VI and consolidated legislation theretofore dispersed in several special education statutes. The EHA also authorized, in Part C, Regional Resource Centers (Section 621); Early Childhood Projects (Section 623), which had originally been authorized by the Handicapped Children's Early Education Assistance Act in 1968; Severely Handicapped Projects (Section 624); and Centers and Services for Deaf-Blind Children (Section 622) (Trudeau, 1971).

STRENGTHENING THE LEGISLATIVE FOUNDATIONS FOR GROWTH: 1970–75

Developmental Disabilities

In 1970, the Developmental Disabilities Services and Facilities Construction Act (PL 91-517) expanded the scope and purpose of PL 88-164 by extending services for the first time to individuals with cerebral palsy and epilepsy. Although the introduction of the statutory concept of "developmental disability" was a distinguishing feature of the 1970 law, perhaps its most important characteristic was the emphasis on coordinated planning and service delivery through a new state formula grant program. To receive formula grant funds, states were required to establish "councils" to develop plans that integrated the proposed activities of several key agencies of state government as they pertained to the delivery of developmental disabilities services. Composition of the state councils established under the act had to include representation from agencies such as public aid/public welfare, education, public health, rehabilitation, and mental health. State developmental disability plans also had to incorporate information on 16 types of services considered essential for the proper care and treatment of persons with developmental disabilities (Stedman, 1976).

Litigative Propellants

The ink was hardly dry on PL 91-517 when, in rapid succession, three events accelerated the pace of federal reform and the intensity of federal funding. First, in October, 1971, a consent agreement was reached in a Philadelphia District Court establishing the judicial right of institutionalized children with mental retardation to a free public education at the expense of the Commonwealth of Pennsylvania (*Pennsylvania Association for Retarded Citizens v. Commonwealth of Pennsylvania*, 1972). Second, only a few months later, Federal Judge Frank M. Johnson ordered sweeping reforms at Alabama's Partlow State School and Hospital (*Wyatt v. Stickney*, 1972). Third, and in quiet contrast, legislation in the fall of 1971 was introduced in the U.S. Senate calling for the U.S. government to pay for part of the excess costs of educating all handicapped children in the nation. This bill, introduced as S.6, was to become PL 94-142, the Education for All Handicapped Children Act of 1975. (For additional discussion of the role of litigation during 1971–75 in expanding educational and related services to persons with disabilities, see Gilhool, 1976; Herr, 1983, 1984; and Herr, Arons, & Wallace, 1983.)

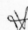

ICF/MR Services

In a fourth watershed event, Congress amended Title XIX of the Social Security Act in December, 1971, permitting state mental retardation institutions, or portions thereof, to receive reimbursements as ICFs/MR. The new program, authorized by PL 92-223, took effect January 1, 1972, and required ICFs/MR to provide "active treatment." Four months later, 28 states had filed amended state Medic-

aid plans with the DHEW Secretary and were participating in the new program. (Wyoming and Arizona are the only two states today that do not participate in the ICF/MR Program.) No one thought it possible at the time, but reimbursements for ICF/MR services have become the largest federally financed mental retardation program.

Rehabilitation Act Strengthened

Expiration of the Vocational Rehabilitation Act in 1972 provided advocates with yet another opportunity to advance the interests of persons with disabilities. Two successful legislative strategies were adopted. First, Congress was pressed to stipulate a priority in rehabilitation services provided to severely disabled persons by state rehabilitation agencies. This priority was mandated in PL 93-112, the Rehabilitation Act of 1973. Agency records indicated that only 7% of all persons with MR/DD rehabilitated in FY 1972 were severely retarded. The share reached 10% in FY 1975, and it remained at that level through FY 1982, declining to 7.9% in FY 1984.

The Rehabilitation Act of 1973 also contained an important civil rights provision prohibiting denial of participation by an "otherwise qualified handicapped individual" in any program or activity receiving federal financial assistance. Regulations issued under this provision, Section 504 of the act, required all federal agencies to promulgate nondiscriminatory regulations. An additional requirement under Section 503 was also adopted, prohibiting employment discrimination by federal contractors (i.e., contractors who had entered into an agreement with the federal government on projects involving more than $2,500).

Due Process in Special Education

The following year, PL 93-380, the Education of the Handicapped Act Amendments of 1974, was enacted. This statute established due process procedural safeguards commonly associated with PL 94-142 (Abeson, Bolick,

& Haas, 1975). Another provision of PL 93-380 authorized PL 89-313 funds to follow relocated children formerly served in state institutions to the community schools they attended. In FY 1984, 39,000 (40%) children with mental retardation receiving services under PL 89-313 were being educated in community settings.

The Education for All Handicapped Children Act of 1975, PL 94-142, greatly expanded the Special Education State Grant Program. Funding doubled from FY 1976 to FY 1977, and again from FY 1978 to FY 1979. The framers intended the act to finance 40% of the excess costs of educating all handicapped children in the United States by FY 1982. In FY 1984, however, funds expended under the program were only an estimated 10% of the excess costs attributable to special education expenditures (Consortium for Citizens with Developmental Disabilities, [Consortium], 1984).

Social Services' Ceiling

Cost controls in the open-end Social Services Program originally authorized by Titles IV and VI of the Social Security Act were legislated in 1972 with the enactment of the State and Local Fiscal Assistance Act (PL 92-512). PL 92-512 froze spending at $2.5 billion annually. The Social Services Program had grown rapidly for a decade, more than doubling between FY 1962 and FY 1972, from $750 million to $1.606 billion. The FY 1974 Social Security Amendments consolidated the Social Services Titles into a new Title XX. Subsequent amendments raised the authorization levels to $2.7 billion (in FY 1976) and to $3.3 billion (in FY 1980).

In FY 1985, however, Congress continued to appropriate only $2.7 billion for the program. The Social Services Program has been an important source of revenue for states and communities developing alternatives to institutional care. In real economic terms, however, services to persons with MR/DD financed with Title XX/Block Grant funds fell 18% between FY 1977 and FY 1984 (Braddock, Hemp, & Howes, 1984).

SSI Authorized

The Supplemental Security Income Program, like the ceiling on Social Services spending, was enacted by the 92nd Congress in 1972. PL 92-603 repealed existing public assistance authorities for persons who were elderly, blind, or disabled and consolidated them into a new Title XVI. Title XVI established a base federal income support level for eligible aged, blind, and disabled persons nationally. Implemented in calendar year 1974, the new SSI Program permitted states to supplement basic SSI payment levels, and it "federalized" administration of the program.

The definition of disability adopted for the SSI Program followed that of the ADC program under Social Security. To be eligible, adult recipients had to have become disabled prior to age 22, and meet a statutory test of severity that precluded "substantial gainful activity." Also, for the first time, children who were disabled became eligible for SSI payments, provided that their disability was comparable in severity to that of adult recipients. About 25% of all disabled recipients of SSI payments in the United States in 1984 were individuals with mental retardation (J. Schmulowitz, personal communication, June 15, 1984).

During the FY 1950–77 period, the SSI Program and its predecessor, Aid to the Permanently and Totally Disabled, were the most heavily funded MR/DD assistance programs sponsored by the federal government. In FY 1984, SSI was providing federal assistance payments to an estimated 588,011 persons with a diagnosis of mental retardation. This figure excludes an additional 42,487 individuals with mental retardation who received SSI State Supplements, but did not receive federal payments.

DIFFUSION AND EXPANSION: 1975–80

The 1975–80 period was characterized by the continuing diffusion of special handicap provisions attached to general purpose social legislation. Educational Aid to Federally Impacted Areas, Small Business Administration Handicapped Assistance Loans, Department of Housing and Urban Development (HUD) Housing Loans, and Food Stamp Assistance were just four of the many programs for which explicit MR/DD support, or general support for all individuals with handicaps, was legislatively stipulated. PL 93-380, the Education of the Handicapped Amendments of 1974, amended the Impact Aid Program by authorizing local educational agencies to receive 150% of their basic per pupil reimbursement for "appropriately served" handicapped children. The 1978 education amendments, PL 95-561, expanded impact aid reimbursement provisions to include handicapped children placed by local school districts into private schools. In FY 1984, impact aid for special education was $64.5 million nationally.

Housing Loans

The 93rd Congress was also responsible for extending the eligible target population for HUD Section 202 Housing Loans, which had first been authorized in 1959, to benefit handicapped individuals. Loans for MR/DD projects under the Housing and Community Development Act of 1974, PL 93-383, were initially approved in FY 1976. In 1977, PL 95-128 required the coordination of Section 202 loan applications with HUD Section 8 Rental Assistance Payments. Amendments enacted in 1978 statutorily mandated that a minimum of $50 million be set aside for housing loans for nonelderly persons with handicaps. By FY 1981, over 60% of the total funding for Section 202–sponsored loans to handicapped individuals was allocated for apartments and group homes for persons who were developmentally disabled or mentally retarded. That year $44.287 million was approved for MR/DD project loans (S. Falconer, U.S. Department of Housing and Urban Development, personal communication, December 4, 1984).

Small Business Loans

Funding for Handicapped Assistance Loans under the Small Business Act Amendments of 1972 was initiated in FY 1974. Under this program, most loans were authorized for nonprofit organizations, including sheltered workshops. Loans have also been made occasionally to businesses owned by handicapped individuals. In FY 1981, $26.9 million was obligated for both types of loans. The Small Business Administration was unable to identify the portion of Handicapped Assistance Loan funds specifically attributable to MR/DD projects.

Food Stamps

Although disabled persons have participated in the Food Stamp Program for many years as ordinary citizens, special provision for this population was not enacted until 1979. That year, PL 96-58 authorized food stamps for persons in community living facilities of less than 16 residents. For the purposes of determining eligibility and monthly coupon allotments, each eligible disabled person was defined as an individual household. Prior to the 1979 legislation, group homes were considered institutions and their residents were ineligible for food stamps (Office for Handicapped Individuals [OHI], 1980).

Developmental Disabilities Act Revisions

During the 1975–80 period, developmental disabilities legislation expired twice and was twice re-enacted in modified form. Expenditure levels envisioned by proponents of the 1970 Developmental Disabilities Services and Facilities Construction Act (PL 91-517) were not reached, although unadjusted spending for the state formula grant program rose from $28.176 million to $43.181 million between FY 1975 and FY 1980. In 1975, PL 91-517 was amended by PL 94-103 to require that states expend at least 30% of their formula grants on deinstitutionalization activities, and that they incorporate deinstitutionalization plans into their state DD plans. Autism was also stipulated in the act as a developmental disability and a new special project grant authority was authorized. UAF support was extended under the legislation. States were also required to develop evaluation plans, but this requirement became controversial and was dropped in subsequent legislation (Braddock, 1977).

PL 94-103 extended the act for 3 years—1975–78. Upon expiration, Congress enacted PL 95-602, the Rehabilitation, Comprehensive Services, and Developmental Disabilities Amendments of 1978. The 1978 legislation significantly revised the definition of a developmental disability. The previous definition—based on the categorical disabilities of mental retardation, cerebral palsy, epilepsy, autism, and dyslexia—was abolished in favor of a "functional" approach. Severity and chronicity remained primary criteria in the revised definition; however, the new definition required the presence of three or more substantial functional limitations in seven areas of major life activity. The seven life activity areas stipulated were self-care, receptive and expressive language, learning, mobility, self-direction, capacity for independent living, and economic self-sufficiency.

PL 95-602 was also notable for instituting a shift of emphasis away from planning to priority services. States were given the option of selecting case management, child development, alternative community living, and/or nonvocational social-developmental services as priorities for the expenditure of state grant funds. The 1978 amendments also authorized establishment of Protection and Advocacy Systems at the state level.

Escalating Expenditures

The diffusion of special provisions for persons with developmental disabilities or mental retardation in general purpose social legislation was accompanied by an unprecedented expansion in the volume of funds expended for previously enacted disability programs. The foundation established during the 1970–75 period in special education (PL 94-142), income maintenance (SSI) and health care (ICF/MR) supported total federal MR/DD expenditures of $2.7 billion in FY 1980. This was an unadjusted increase of more than 200% over the FY 1975 funding level.

THE REAGAN ERA: 1981–

Reconciliation and Austerity

President Ronald Reagan's first month in office in 1981 was marked by the introduction of his "Program for Economic Recovery." Much of the program he proposed was enacted in the Omnibus Budget Reconciliation Act (OBRA) of 1981, PL 97-35. This legislation called for extensive budget cuts in domestic social programs, large multipurpose block grants in lieu of categorical state grant programs, and increased defense spending (Braddock, 1981; Gettings, 1981). Unparalleled in scope, the act reduced previously legislated authorization levels for many domestic programs for FY 1982–84. As a result, there was little or no growth during FY 1981–84 in special education, vocational education, rehabilitation, social services, research and training across the board, and in Developmental Disabilities Act services (Braddock, 1986c; Braddock, Hemp, & Howes, 1985).

Although PL 97-35 provided incentives to states to reduce the rate of growth in Medicaid spending, an expenditure "ceiling" was not legislated per se. The OBRA required that federal Medicaid payments be reduced by 3% in FY 1982, 4% in FY 1983, and 4.5% in FY 1984. (The Reagan Administration proposed a permanent 3.5% annual reduction commencing in FY 1985.) Also notable among the act's Medicaid provisions was the Section 2176 (b) amendment to Section 1915(c)(1) of the Social Security Act, authorizing waivers for "Home and Community-Based Care." In lieu of providing more expensive ICF/MR care in institutions, states were authorized to file amended Medicaid plans for reimbursable services in alternative community settings.

Waivered services included personal and homemaker care, case management services, home health care, habilitation services, and respite care. Room and board costs were excluded. Applicant states had to demonstrate that the cost of providing these alternative services would be less than the cost of institutional care. Waivers have been popular—45

states had obtained 78 approved waivers as of
January 1, 1985 (National Association of
State Mental Retardation Program Directors
[National Association], 1985). Their overall
impact on state MR/DD service systems,
however, has been modest to date (Braddock
et al., 1984). On June 3, 1985, Senators
Bradley, Chiles, and Glenn introduced a bill
(S.1277, 99th Congress, 1st Session) authorizing states to provide home and community
services without the necessity of obtaining a
waiver.

Block Grants

The Title XX Social Services Program authorized by the 1974 Social Security Amendments was converted into a Block Grant
Program under PL 97-35, and states were af-
forded greater flexibility in administration of
the program. State matching funds were no
longer required by the federal government, although some states continued to require local
matching funds of their grantees and vendors.

A new Maternal and Child Health (MCH)
Block Grant was also authorized by PL 97-35,
consolidating funding from Title V programs
in Maternal and Child Health and Crippled
Children's Services State Grants with Lead
Based Paint Poisoning Prevention Grants. A
"15% set-aside" in the MCH Block Grant
stipulated support for Genetic Disease Projects, Regional Hemophilia Diagnostic and
Treatment Centers, Pediatric Pulmonary Centers, applied research, and also Section 511
training conducted at UAFs. Total funding for
MCH services in FY 1981 was $456.7 mil-
lion. Under the Block Grant, funding was
$373 million in the following year, $478 million in FY 1983 (including a $105 million sup-
plemental appropriation), and $399 million in
FY 1984.

The OBRA also established the Alcohol,
Drug Abuse, and Mental Health (ADM)
Block Grant, with about half of the funding
authorized therein designated for community
mental health services and half for substance
abuse services. Up to 15% of the funds could
be transferred at the state's discretion between

the two programs. Funds appropriated for the
ADM Block Grant totaled $432 million for
FY 1982, $468 million for FY 1983, and $462
million for FY 1984. This compares to the FY
1981 funding level for community mental
health, exclusive of substance abuse funds, of
$326 million (Consortium, 1984). Thus,
block grants brought the states more flexible
administration and less money in the areas of
Social Services, health care, and mental
health (U.S. General Accounting Office
[GAO], 1982).

Special Education and Vocational Rehabilitation

There were few changes in Special Education
and Vocational Rehabilitation legislation during President Reagan's first term. However,
amendments were enacted revising each program slightly in 1983 and 1984.

Developmental Disabilities Act Amendments of 1984

The 1978 Developmental Disabilities Act
Amendments (PL 95-602) expired in 1981,
and provisions were included in the OBRA
(PL 97-35) that extended the basic legislation.
Three years later, the Developmental Disabilities Act Amendments of 1984 became
law. The "purposes" section of the act was
amended in Part A, Section 101, to include
assisting states to "ensure that developmentally disabled persons will receive the services
necessary for them to achieve their maximum
potential through increased independence,
productivity, and integration into the community." The 1984 amendments redefined priority services to include employment-related
activities and deleted nonvocational social-
developmental services as a priority. The
amendments required states to include
employment-related activities as priority services for any fiscal year after FY 1986 for
which the total appropriation for state grants is
at least $50.25 million. The Secretary of
Health and Human Services was also required
to establish standards for UAFs (U.S. House
of Representatives [House], 1984).

FY 1985 Appropriations Rebound

FY 1985 appropriations for social programs rebounded somewhat from the unprecedented across-the-board cutbacks dictated by the OBRA. Developmental Disabilities State Grants, for example, advanced from $43.75 million in FY 1984, to $50.25 million. This was the first significant increase in formula grant funds since FY 1980. Funding for Protection and Advocacy jumped from $8.4 to $13.7 million. There were slight increases in the state grant programs for Special Education and Vocational Rehabilitation in FY 1985 as well. These programs advanced from $1.068 to $1.135 billion and from $1.038 to $1.118 billion, respectively. Advocates for persons with disabilities could also point to other achievements at the close of President Reagan's first term. Although several important categorical programs had been "blocked," PL 94-142 had not, nor had the Developmental Disabilities and Vocational Rehabilitation Programs.

Disability Benefits Reform

On October 9, 1984, the president signed into law the Social Security Disability Benefits Reform Act of 1984. This legislation amended Title II of the Social Security Act, prohibiting the termination of disability benefits unless there was "evidence of medical improvement in the individual's impairment," and the individual became able to engage in substantial gainful activity (SGA). An advancement in diagnosis, therapy, or technology providing the beneficiary with the ability to perform SGA was also defined as justifiable grounds for termination, as was the ability of the beneficiary to perform SGA as a consequence of vocational therapy.

This legislation was a particularly important achievement because of a major controversy in 1982–83 associated with the termination of benefits for tens of thousands of Title II disability beneficiaries. Congress had authorized a review of the disability rolls in 1980. During the Reagan administration's subsequent im-

plementation, approximately 490,000 persons, or about 40% of the 1.2 million cases that had been reviewed, were terminated. About half of the beneficiaries who appealed termination decisions had their benefits restored. An alarmed Congress took up the issue in the spring of 1984. The Social Security Disability Benefits Reform Act of 1984 was the result.

Under the new act, benefit payments continued during eligibility appeals, but if the decision was adverse to the individual, benefits had to be repaid to the government. A moratorium was also initiated for all disability cases involving mental impairment until the applicable criteria could be revised by the Social Security Administration. Reimbursements paid to state vocational rehabilitation agencies for their costs incurred while serving disability beneficiaries were also partially reinstated. Finally, if eligible beneficiaries recovered medically while receiving rehabilitation services, such services were now reimbursable. PL 97-35 had previously stipulated that disability beneficiaries had to work at SGA for 9 months for rehabilitation services to be reimbursable (National Association of State Mental Retardation Program Directors [National Association], 1984).

Baby Doe

As President Reagan's first term drew to a close, Congress also passed disability legislation in another controversial area—that of "Baby Doe." The President signed the Child Abuse Amendments of 1984 (PL 98-457) on the same day he inscribed the Disability Reform Amendments. PL 98-457 contained a provision inhibiting the withholding of medical treatment from infants born with mental and physical disabilities. State child protection agencies were required to establish procedures for responding to reports that disabled newborns were being denied "medically indicated treatment." Treatment was required unless: 1) the infant was irreversibly comatose; 2) treatment would merely prolong dying or not ameliorate all life-threatening conditions;

or 3) treatment was futile. To pay for the new disabled infant provisions, Congress increased authorizations under the Child Abuse and Neglect Act (PL 93-247, as Amended) by $5 million in FY 1984–87. The new legislation also authorized the establishment of national and regional information clearinghouses.

SUMMARY AND CONCLUSION

The evolution of federal assistance programs for mental retardation and developmental disabilities during the preceding 25 years has been summarized in this chapter. The review covered the period from the issuance of the report of the President's Panel on Mental Retardation (President's Panel, 1962) through the enactment of the Developmental Disabilities Act Amendments of 1984. During this period, annual federal spending for MR/DD programs grew from $118 million to $7.773 billion.

Many of the most important recommendations of the President's Panel were enacted into law by the 88th Congress as PL 88-156 and PL 88-164. The latter act authorized the construction of UAFs, Research Centers, and Community Facilities. Broad-based growth in federal MR/DD programs after 1965 was stimulated through congressional earmarks and special eligibility provisions attached to Great Society enactments.

During the seventies, the concept of developmental disabilities was introduced into law. New or greatly expanded programs were established in SSI, food stamps, Social Services, rehabilitation of severe disability, housing loans, and civil rights protections. The unprecedented expansion of health and special education services was authorized with the passage of the Medicaid ICF/MR amendment in 1971, and, four years later, of PL 94-142.

The Reagan administration curtailed federal spending for social programs, and transformed certain categorical programs in public health and Social Services into administratively flexible block grants. As the president's first term drew to a close, two vital concerns of advocates for persons with disabilities were: to what extent would the administration be able to repeat its remarkable "Omnibus" accomplishments of 1981; and, to what extent could it subdue escalating entitlement programs in health care and Social Security.

There was little doubt in early 1985 that the new administration would try for a repeat performance as the deficit soared beyond the $200 billion mark. Now, in this austere context, the most important issue of the 99th Congress turns on the fate of the revised version of S.2053, the Community and Family Living Amendments. The revised bill, S.873, sponsored by Senator John Chafee, proposes to redirect federal ICF/MR support from state-operated institutions to small, community-based alternatives.

Chapters 3–8 of this volume probe beyond the historical review presented in Chapters 1 and 2, and further analyze underlying financial trends in much greater depth. The utility of investigations of the type presented in this book has increased significance in times of fiscal austerity, and during periods of fundamental reconsideration of financial policy. Such are the times in mental retardation and developmental disabilities.

PART II

ANALYTICAL PROFILES
OF FEDERAL PROGRAMS

Chapter 3

Services Programs

THE "SERVICES" CATEGORY contains the largest number (36) of individual MR/DD program elements identified in the six classification categories employed in the federal analysis component of the MR/DD Expenditure Analysis Project. The 36 services program elements represent two-thirds of all 53 currently active elements in FY 1985 identified in this study. In FY 1977, federal funding for services first surpassed income maintenance payments as the highest funded MR/DD activity at the federal level. Since that date, the margin of expenditure for services over income maintenance payments has widened every year. This has principally been due to the rapid growth of three large programs: the Title XIX program of intermediate care facilities for the mentally retarded (ICFs/MR), PL 94-142 Special Education State Grants, and the Noninstitutional Medicaid Program that provides health care services to MR/DD community residents.

MR/DD services include the following four components: 1) *Educational Services,* which is further subdivided into special education, vocational education, and impact aid; 2) *Vocational Rehabilitation Services,* primarily state grants; 3) *Public Health Services,* which includes, among other Department of Health and Human Services (DHHS) programs, ICF/MR, noninstitutional Medicaid, Medicare, and Department of Defense activities; and 4) *Human Development Services,* consisting of Developmental Disabilities Act services, social services, and volunteer services. Federal funding for services in FY 1985 is depicted in Figure 2.

The growth of federal financing for services is divisible into three historical periods. The post–World War II era, 1945–61, begins with the initial implementation in the states of amendments to the Vocational Rehabilitation Act authorizing eligibility for mentally handicapped clients. It embraces Congressman Fogarty's initiatives in 1955, and it concludes with the appointment of President Kennedy's panel on mental retardation. The second historical period, 1962–71, commences with the issuance of the panel's recommendations in 1962, and it includes the subsequent implementation of many of those recommendations in the laws enacted by the 88th Congress. It concludes with President Richard M. Nixon's November 16, 1971, "Statement on Mental Retardation" (White House, 1971). That statement pledged "continuing expansion" of the growing federal commitment to mental retardation, and it stipulated major national goals in prevention and deinstitutionalization.

The third historical period, 1972–85, commences with the January, 1972, implementation of PL 92-223. This law embodied the amendments first authorizing federal intermediate care facility disbursements to state institutions providing "active treatment" to mentally retarded individuals (ICFs/MR). The third historical period includes the subsequent expansion of federal funding for ICF/MR reimbursed services, for PL 94-142 Special Education State Grants, and for SSI. It includes funds budgeted during the first term of President Ronald Reagan. Figures 3, 4, and 5 depict the growth of federal expenditures for services in the three historical periods.

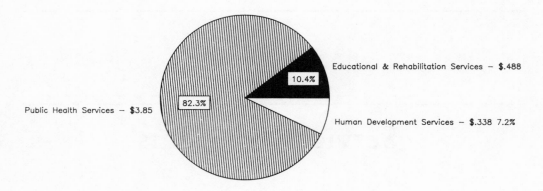

Total: $4.676 Billion

Figure 2.   Federal support for MR/DD services: FY 1985. (Dollars are in billions).

In real economic terms, total federal funding for services has increased annually every year since FY 1954. In FY 1981, however, the rate of that growth slowed appreciably. Real growth during FY 1981–85 totaled 5.4%, or an average of 2.2% annually. This contrasts with an average rate of real economic growth from FY 1972 to FY 1980 of 15.5% per year. The greatly reduced real growth rate since 1981 is primarily attributa-

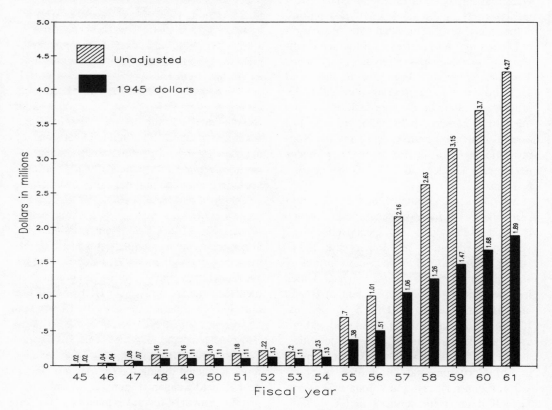

Figure 3.   Federal expenditures for MR/DD services: FY 1945–61.

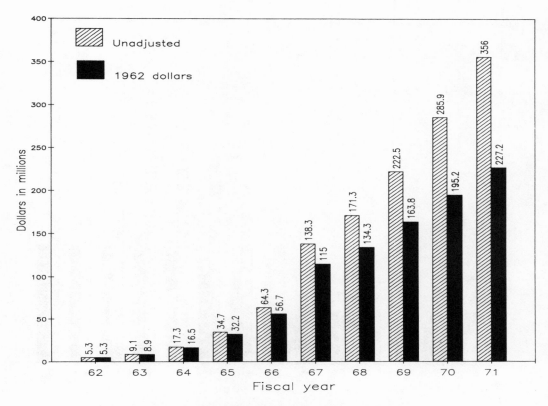

Figure 4.   Federal expenditures for MR/DD services: FY 1962–71.

ble to the diminished rate of growth in federal ICF/MR reimbursements. Federal ICF/MR payments were projected to actually decline slightly in real economic terms between FY 1984 and FY 1985.

Although the overall trends in federal spending for MR/DD services move steadily upward, from FY 1972 to FY 1985, this global trend conceals quite diverse funding patterns for individual programs. The following discussion describes federal expenditures for each individual program under these services subcategories: 1) educational services; 2) vocational rehabilitation services; 3) public health services; and 4) human development services. Each program discussion contains: 1) a detailed profile of the program; 2) a table displaying the MR/DD expenditures and other program data when available; 3) the source of the data; and 4) for major programs, a discussion of the expenditure trends over the history of the program.

EDUCATIONAL SERVICES

The domestic educational services mission of the federal government most relevant to the needs of persons with MR/DD consists of three types of activities: 1) special education services; 2) vocational education services; and 3) impact aid to federally affected schools. In FY 1985, the large majority of funds budgeted for services to children and youth with mental retardation were allocated under the auspices of the special education programs, as illustrated in Figure 6.

Special Education

PL 89-313, Title I/Chapter I: Aid to State Schools Funds to state-operated or state-supported schools for the operation of educational programs for handicapped children throughout the United States are provided under this program. Local education agencies also may participate in the program on behalf

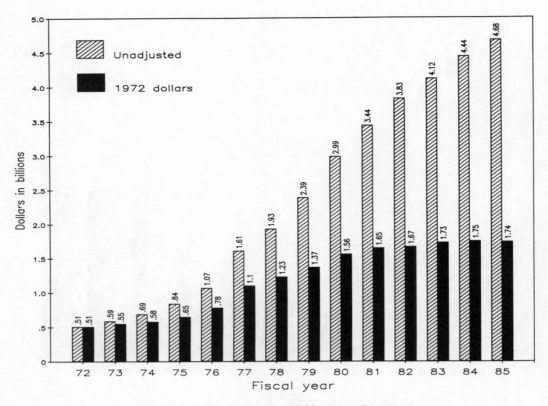

Figure 5. Federal expenditures for MR/DD services: FY 1972–85.

of deinstitutionalized children formerly residing in state institutions. Funds are used to provide classroom instruction, physical education, mobility training, counseling, prevocational and vocational education, teacher training, and training for teachers' aides. In FY 1984, an estimated 97,452 of 247,291 handicapped children who participated in the program were mentally retarded; this represented a drop from 59% of all children served

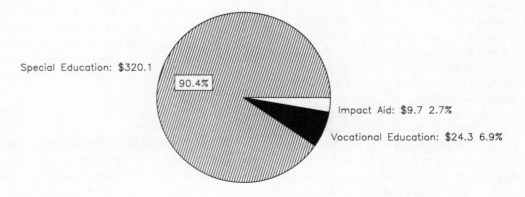

Special Education: $320.1

90.4%

Impact Aid: $9.7 2.7%

Vocational Education: $24.3 6.9%

Total: $354.1 Million

Figure 6. Educational services to children and youth with mental retardation: FY 1985. (Dollars are in millions.)

in FY 1970–73 to 39% in 1984. The number of children with mental retardation served has fallen from a high of 120,204 in FY 1978, to 97,452 in FY 1984. However, although the number of retarded children participating in the program has dropped steadily in recent years, the number of deinstitutionalized children "followed" to local school systems increased from about 7,000 to more than 39,000 between FY 1975 and FY 1982.

PL 89-313 was enacted in 1965, several months after the passage of the landmark Elementary and Secondary Education Act (ESEA). Title I of ESEA had authorized a billion dollar program of federal aid to local school districts for the provision of educational services to educationally "disadvantaged" children. States were initially entitled to receive PL 89-313 funding on the basis of the number of eligible handicapped children multiplied by the state average per capita expenditure for all children enrolled in elementary and secondary schools. PL 90-247, enacted in 1967, mandated "full funding" for the program and it established funding on the basis of either the state or the national average per pupil expenditure, whichever was higher.

The Education of the Handicapped Amendments of 1974, PL 93-380, revised the program's funding formula, causing relatively more funds to be deployed to southern and rural areas and less to large cities and relatively wealthy states. PL 93-380 also authorized follow-through educational funding for children who were relocated from state institutions to community settings. In such cases, the state agency could continue counting these children for purposes of the PL 89-313 funding formula, but it was required to forward funds received to the local educational agencies actually providing the services to the children. PL 93-380 also protected PL 89-313 appropriations from future cutbacks under the newly adopted ESEA Title I formula.

The 1978 revisions to PL 89-313 brought it into closer conformity with the state grant program authorized under Part B of the Education of the Handicapped Act (PL 91-230, Title VI). In 1981, the Education Consolidation and

Table 2. PL 89-313, aid to children in state schools, mental retardation funding history: FY 1966–1985 (dollars are in thousands)

FY	Children with mental retardation served	Mental retardation obligations
1966		$8,354
1967		$8,473
1968		$13,685
1969	63,605	$16,543
1970		$21,664
1971		$26,929
1972		$32,826
1973	98,760	$46,900
1974	103,000	$52,500
1975	111,600	$54,828
1976	113,000	$57,633
1977	118,000	$59,084
1978	120,204	$61,377
1979	114,260	$62,134
1980	112,899	$60,147
1981	111,381	$56,522
1982	103,835	$62,606
1983	102,777	$61,281
1984	97,452	$57,728
1985	97,452	$59,166

Source: Data for FY 1966–72 are from Braddock (1973, p. 59). Data for FY 1973–76 are from House appropriations subcommittee supplementary data (OHI, 1976, p. 13). The source of FY 1977–84 data is: Administrative Records, Budget Office, Office of Special Education, U.S. Department of Education, (M. Abramson, personal communications, November 23, 1983; June, 1984; October 22, 1984; and November 20, 1984; B. Wolfe, personal communication, August 19, 1983). Mental retardation spending data were imputed from the actual numbers of children with mental retardation receiving services. Estimated cost data for FY 1985 were imputed from the 1984 pupil count and FY 1985 appropriation for ESEA Chapter I (PL 89-313).

Improvement Act revised PL 89-313's funding formula by redesignating it as "Chapter I" and establishing a fiscal ceiling. The act capped state school funding at 14.6% of total Chapter I appropriations in conjunction with all the special Chapter I state fundings, such as migrant and dependent/neglected aid. (See Table 2 for the numbers of children served by PL 89-313 and the amount of money spent during FY 1966–1985.)

Prior to the implementation of PL 94-142, PL 89-313 was the largest program of educational assistance to handicapped or mentally retarded children in the United States. Federal spending for children with mental retardation

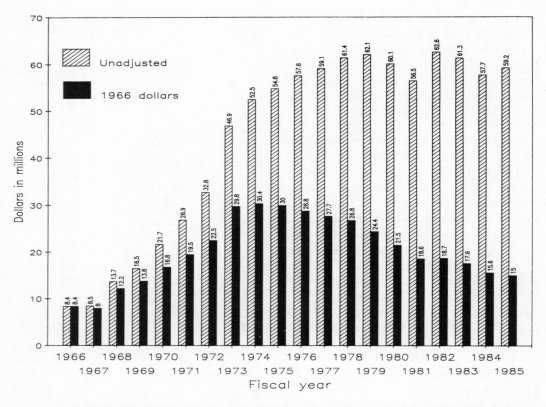

Figure 7.   PL 89-313, aid to children in state schools, mental retardation funding history: FY 1966–85.

grew every year from FY 1966 to FY 1979, advancing from $8.4 million to $62.1 million, respectively. From FY 1979 to FY 1985, the program leveled off. The appropriation for FY 1985 was $59.2 million, down 4.8% from the FY 1979 figure on an unadjusted basis (see Figure 7).

In adjusted terms, the program's funding grew steadily during FY 1966–74. From FY 1975 to FY 1985, funding declined just as steadily by a total factor of 50% over the entire decade. During this later period, the population of persons of all ages residing in state mental retardation institutions declined nearly as much. Between FY 1977 and FY 1984, according to the survey conducted in preparation of the present volume, the institutional population dropped 26.6%, from 149,535 to 109,827.

ESEA, Title II: Aid to State School Libraries The Library Services and Construction Act (LSCA) Amendment of 1966 revised the original Library Act of 1957 by authorizing a program of assistance to states for providing library services in state mental institutions, prisons, and other similar special residential facilities. Under Title I of the LSCA, funds were deployed based on state plans and could be used for the acquisition of books and library materials, equipment, salaries, and administrative expenses. Sixty-five MR/DD institutions received small grants in FY 1975. Total funds expended in MR/DD institutions on a nationwide basis ranged between $27,000 and $80,000 during FY 1968–76. Data specific to MR/DD institutions have not been gathered on a nationwide basis since FY 1976.

PL 94-142, Title VI, Part B: State Grants The Special Education State Grant Program was initially authorized by Title VI of PL 89-750 in 1967. This was the same law that created the Bureau of Education for the Handicapped in the U.S. Office of Education. The bureau was the forerunner of today's Office of Special Education and Rehabilitative Services in the U.S. Department of Education. The program was modestly funded for several years after enactment. Total spending under Title VI, Part B, in fact, did not exceed $37.5 million until FY 1974. The ESEA Amendments of 1970, PL 91-230, consolidated several separate special education statutes, including Part B, into a single Title VI. Title VI has been commonly referred to as the "Education of the Handicapped Act."

Amendments in 1974, PL 93-380, authorized a large increase in state grants and Part B funding reached $100 million in FY 1976. The 1974 amendments had other key features marking it as landmark legislation in the field. It required states to establish a goal of and plan for providing "full educational opportunities" for "all" handicapped children; and

it simultaneously provided for procedural safeguards for identification, evaluation, and placement of handicapped children, encouraging placement in regular classes when possible. The act also elevated the head of the Bureau of Education for the Handicapped to the position of Deputy Commissioner of Education.

PL 94-142 was enacted in 1975, and expanded state grant funding from a quite small program into a commitment on a scale with the large federal presence in the programs of Vocational Education and Education of Disadvantaged Children. Between FY 1976 and FY 1977, total funding for Part B doubled. By 1979, it had almost tripled—to $563.9 million (see Figure 8 and Figure 9). It nearly doubled again by 1984, when it surpassed $1 billion. It should be noted, however, that as the act was originally written, it was to assume, over a several year period, 40% of the national average per pupil expenditure for educating all

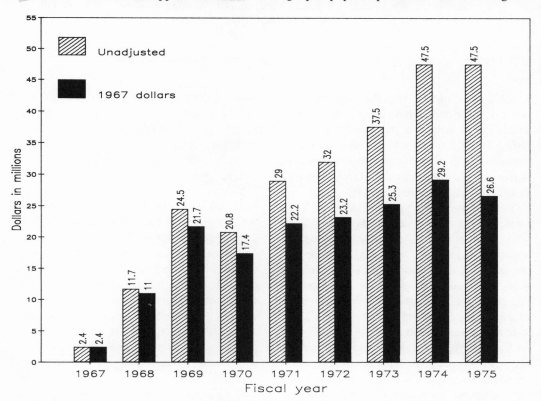

Figure 8. Title VI B Special Education State Grants for all handicapped children: FY 1967–75.

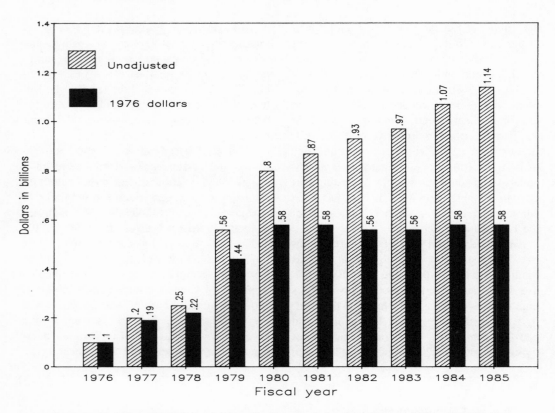

Figure 9.   PL 94-142, Title VI B Special Education State Grants for all handicapped children: FY 1976–85.

handicapped children. Had this been the case in FY 1984, it would have been generating in excess of $4 billion in federal funds. In FY 1984, Part B funding actually represented an estimated 10% of per pupil costs nationwide (Consortium for Citizens with Developmental Disabilities [Consortium], 1984).

The purpose of the Special Education State Grant Program is to assist states and local schools in providing specially designed instruction and related services to meet the unique needs of a handicapped child. Related services include: transportation, developmental, corrective, and other supportive services to assist a handicapped child to benefit from special education. Part B funds are allocated on the basis of a statutory formula based on the state's count of handicapped children served therein. PL 94-142 called for a gradually escalating percentage of federal aid beginning with 5% of the average per pupil expen-

diture in the United States to 40% in FY 1982 and thereafter. However, the Omnibus Budget Reconciliation Act (OBRA) of 1981 contained language superseding the statutory funding formula in PL 94-142 and dramatically slowed fiscal growth (see Table 3).

The instructional centerpiece of the state grant program is the requirement that all children served must have an individualized education program (IEP) and this program must be reviewed at least annually. The IEP must include a statement of the child's current educational performance, short-term instructional objectives and annual goals, a description of services to be provided, and a statement of anticipated participation in regular education programs. To receive funds under the act, local school systems and intermediate units must submit an approved application to their state education agency.

PL 94-142 also extended and strengthened

Table 3. Estimated PL 94-142, Title VI B Special Education State Grant Program spending attributable to mental retardation: FY 1967–1985 (dollars are in thousands)

FY	Total obligations	% MR students	Cost factor	Estimated MR obligations
1967	$2,425	44.00%	1.4	$1,494
1968	$11,700	44.00%	1.4	$7,207
1969	$24,500	37.00%	1.4	$12,691
1970	$20,800	39.00%	1.4	$11,357
1971	$29,000	33.00%	1.4	$13,398
1972	$32,000	31.00%	1.4	$13,888
1973	$37,500	28.18%	1.4	$14,795
1974	$47,500	27.15%	1.4	$18,055
1975	$47,500	26.11%	1.4	$17,363
1976	$100,000	25.07%	1.4	$35,098
1977	$200,000	24.05%	1.4	$67,340
1978	$253,837	23.15%	1.4	$82,269
1979	$563,875	21.76%	1.4	$171,779
1980	$803,956	20.22%	1.4	$227,596
1981	$874,500	18.63%	1.4	$228,087
1982	$931,008	17.50%	1.4	$228,097
1983	$970,000	16.73%	1.4	$227,193
1984	$1,068,875	15.95%	1.4	$238,680
1985	$1,135,145	14.99%	1.4	$238,222

Source: The Office of Special Education (OSE) does not gather state grant expenditure information specific to individual disabilities; however, data are collected by the OSE annually on the numbers of children served in each disability category. This year's "child count" in fact, becomes the basis of next year's state formula grant allotments. In FY 1982, 17.5% of all handicapped children served were mentally retarded, and the OSE obligated $931.008 million for the total State Grant Program. Based on Kakalik, Furry, Thomas, and Carney's study (1981) of the relative cost of educational services for the various handicaps, educating a child with MR/DD is approximately 40% more expensive than educating the "average" handicapped child. Therefore, the formula used to calculate estimated MR/DD expenditures for FY 1982, as an example, is 17.5% × $931.008 million × 1.4 = $228.097 million.

The source of child count data is an OSE Data Analysis System (DANS) (M. Abramson, personal communication, August 23, 1984). The FY 1985 MR percentage of the total child count was estimated by reducing the FY 1984 percentage by the same factor as the percentage decrease from FY 1983 to FY 1984. Expenditure data for the total State Grant Program were also furnished by Abramson (personal communication, August 23, 1984) for FY 1977–85. Bill Wolfe, OSE Budget Officer, provided total expenditure figures for FY 1973–77 (personal communication, August 19, 1983). Historical expenditure and child data for FY 1967–72 are from Braddock (1973, p. 44).

the due process safeguards set forth in PL 93-380. Additional rights were stipulated, including the following parent/guardian requirements: 1) the opportunity to examine all relevant educational records; 2) written notice of identification, evaluation, or placement; and 3) an opportunity to present complaints, and to do so represented by counsel in the context of an impartial due process hearing conducted by the state/local agency.

Since FY 1967, the percentage of children with mental retardation identified in the annual child count has fallen steadily. The percentage has dropped from a high of 44% in FY 1967, to 15% in FY 1985 (see Figure 10). In absolute terms, however, the number of retarded children actually served under PL 94-142 has fallen from 838,083 in FY 1977 to 653,010 in FY 1984. A primary reason for the fall in the share of children with mental retardation served has been the implementation of educational assistance to children with "learning disabilities." Some children who might have been formerly classified as mildly retarded are being served in this new category.

Estimated spending for PL 94-142 services to children with mental retardation rose on an unadjusted basis steadily from FY 1967 to 1974. Funding skyrocketed in FY 1976–79, remained flat for FY 1980–83, increased 5% in FY 1984, and was essentially unchanged in FY 1985. In real economic terms, however, mental retardation funding peaked in FY 1980 and fell steadily every year thereafter through FY 1985. Mental retardation funds budgeted in FY 1985 were 25% below the FY 1980 level on an adjusted basis. These trends are depicted in Figure 11 and Figure 12.

PL 94-142, Title VI, Part B: Preschool Incentive Grants PL 94-142 contains a provision to encourage states and localities to expand early intervention services to very young handicapped children. The funding formula provides an incentive to participating jurisdictions. Recipients are entitled to $300 times the number of handicapped children age 3–5 being served. (A recent count identified 242,104 children.) This would be sufficient to generate about three times the funds actually

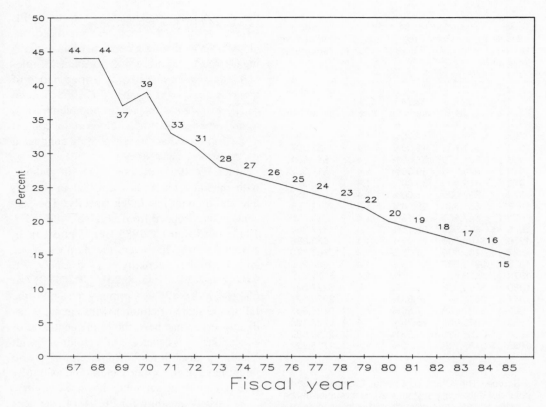

Figure 10.   Nationwide percentage of children with mental retardation identified in annual child counts under PL 94-142:
FY 1967–85.

appropriated for the program in FY 1984. (See Table 4 for a breakdown of the dollars appropriated under the program for children with MR/DD.)

Funds appropriated by Congress have always been substantially less than the numbers generated by the incentive child count formula. (See Figure 13 for the funding history.) In 1984, Congress enacted the Education of the Handicapped Act Amendments, PL 98-199. This legislation contained several provisions strengthening early intervention provisions, among them a clause extending children's eligibility downward, to birth–5 years instead of 3–5 years.

PL 91-230, Title VI, Parts C and F: Special Programs   Public Law 91-230, Title VI C, authorized four small programs that provide highly specialized services and technical assistance for handicapped children and

Table 4.   PL 94-142 Preschool Incentive Grants: FY 1977–85 (dollars are in thousands)

FY	Total $	% MR/DD	Estimated MR/DD $
1977	$12,500	24.05%	$4,209
1978	$15,000	23.15%	$4,862
1979	$17,500	21.76%	$5,331
1980	$25,000	20.22%	$7,077
1981	$25,000	18.63%	$6,521
1982	$24,000	17.50%	$5,880
1983	$25,000	16.73%	$5,856
1984	$26,330	15.95%	$5,879
1985	$29,000	14.99%	$6,086

Source: Figures on total spending were obtained from the OSE Budget Office (B. Wolfe, personal communication, August 19, 1983). A 1.4 cost factor was not used, however, because fewer of the "less expensive" handicaps such as speech impairment and learning disability are identified and, therefore, served in children age 3–5. The cost of educating a child with mental retardation is assumed to be no more or no less than educating the average handicapped child served.

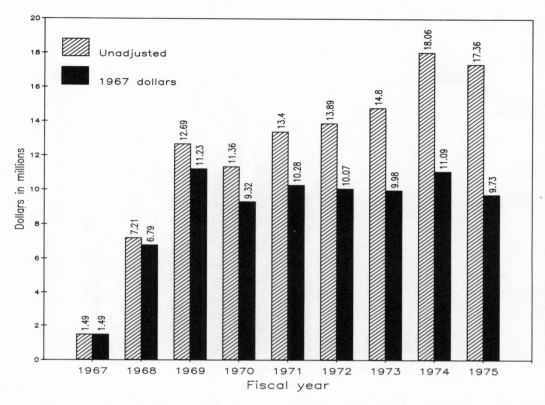

Figure 11.   PL 94-142, Title VI B estimated Special Education State Grant spending for mental retardation: FY 1967–75.

youth. *Regional Resource Centers,* originally authorized in 1967 by PL 90-247, provide advice and technical assistance to special and regular educators on improving the quality of instructional and related services to handicapped children. The centers are located in higher education institutions and state education agencies.

Early Childhood Projects were initially authorized under PL 90-538, the Handicapped Children's Early Education Assistance Act, and reframed as Title VI C, Section 623 of PL 91-230. This is a project grant program, supporting experimental demonstration projects. The network of projects is commonly referred to as the "First Chance Network," and has been responsible for pioneering many new instructional techniques and intervention strategies with preschool children.

Severely Handicapped Projects are supported under Section 624 of PL 91-230, as Amended. The purpose of the projects is to demonstrate innovative approaches to improving educational services to severely handicapped children. *Centers for Deaf-Blind Children* (Part C, Section 622) are responsible for providing highly specialized services to deaf-blind children on a regional basis throughout the United States, including: 1) comprehensive diagnostic and evaluative services; 2) a program of education; and 3) consultation with parents, teachers, and others involved in the child's welfare. PL 90-247 is the original authorization for the Severely Handicapped Projects Program and for Centers for Deaf-Blind Children.

Instructional Media (Part F) is primarily a program providing instructional assistance, such as captioned films, for deaf individuals. The program, however, has historically supported a few special projects on curriculum development, teacher training, and research in

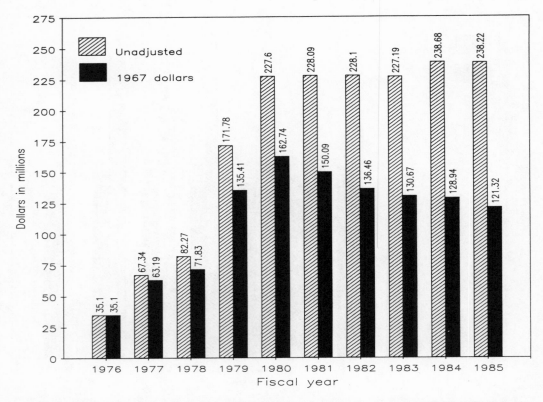

Figure 12.   PL 94-142, Title VI B estimated Special Education State Grant spending for mental retardation: FY 1976–85.

the use of media that pertained to children with mental retardation and developmental disabilities.

In summary, children with MR/DD are participating in these special programs to varying degrees. The greatest level of participation is in the Deaf-Blind Centers Program, where more than half of the children served have mental retardation or other developmental disabilities, and in the Severely Handicapped Projects Program. Children with MR/DD are probably benefiting from Regional Resource Center operations and Early Childhood Projects in approximate accord with their numbers among the general population of handicapped school children. MR/DD participation in the Instructional Media Program is modest, but historically important. (Table 5 shows the total funding for the programs of Title VI Parts C and F and the estimated funding attributable to children with MR/DD.)

Vocational Education

PL 90-576 as Amended: State Grants   Vocational education activities sponsored by the federal government were first authorized in 1917, under the Smith-Hughes Act. This was the first program of "grants-in-aid" to all states in the field of public health, education, and welfare. In 1963, a major enactment, PL 88-210, authorized funds for the construction of vocational schools, work study programs, and demonstration programs. Handicapped children and youth were authorized to participate in the program, but participation was very limited. Braddock (1973, p. 64) reported that only .2% of the program's funding was expended on services to handicapped children.

In 1968, Congress enacted legislation, PL 90-576, amending the Vocational Education Act, requiring that 10% of the funds expended under the state grant program had to be spent

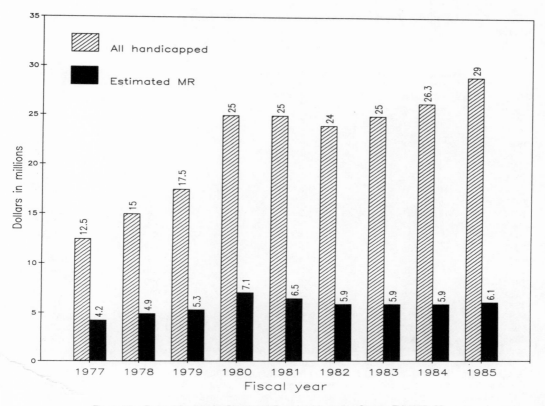

Figure 13.   Federal funding for PL 94-142 Preschool Incentive Grants: FY 1977–85.

for services to children with handicaps. The Education Amendments of 1976, PL 94-482, extended the 10% earmark and raised state matching funds requirements for handicap programs to 50%. The act also encouraged the integration of students with handicaps into regular vocational education programs and classes; and it required that Part B state grant funds authorized under PL 90-576 be expended in conformity with the state's plan filed under provisions of PL 94-142.

In unadjusted terms, spending for mental retardation services grew rapidly during FY 1965–73, essentially paralleling the growth of total state grant appropriations and of obligations for all handicapped youth. It was FY 1971, however, before 10% of the total state grant funds budgeted were expended for services to handicapped youth. Mental retardation funding leveled off for 2 years, FY 1973–74, surged 14% in 1975 and then plunged

39% over the next 3 years. It resumed a steady annual growth rate of 6.6% per year from FY 1979 to FY 1984, and was projected to increase slightly again in FY 1985. (See Table 6.)

In real economic terms, funding for services to youth with mental retardation rose steadily and peaked in FY 1973. Real spending declined by 53%, however, between FY 1973 and FY 1978. Since then, funding has leveled off, with the FY 1984 real spending level being the same as it was in FY 1978. Funding in FY 1985 was projected to decline another 3% in real economic terms. Vocational education spending for persons with mental retardation fell by a total of 55% during FY 1973–85. These trends are depicted in Figure 14.

The budgetary trends in mental retardation spending reflected in Figure 14 were generally reflected in the overall expenditure pattern for

Table 5.   Estimated special education funding for Title VI, Parts C and F, PL 91-230 as Amended (dollars are in thousands)

FY	Regional Resource Centers: Total funding	Regional Resource Centers: MR funding	Early Childhood Projects: Total funding	Early Childhood Projects: MR funding
1966				
1967				
1968				
1969		$185	$945	$349
1970		$1,170	$4,000	$1,560
1971		$984	$7,000	$2,310
1972		$1,101	$7,500	$2,325
1973		$2,028	$12,000	$3,381
1974	$9,691	$2,631	$12,000	$3,259
1975	$9,691	$2,530	$14,000	$3,655
1976	$9,691	$2,430	$22,000	$5,515
1977	$9,388	$2,258	$22,000	$5,291
1978	$9,748	$2,257	$22,000	$5,093
1979	$9,748	$2,121	$22,000	$4,787
1980	$9,748	$1,971	$20,000	$4,044
1981	$7,655	$1,426	$17,500	$3,260
1982	$2,876	$503	$16,800	$2,940
1983	$4,128	$691	$16,800	$2,811
1984	$5,700	$909	$21,100	$3,365
1985	$6,000	$899	$22,500	$3,373

Source: Regional Resource Center total expenditure data for FY 1974–85 were obtained from the OSE Budget Office (B. Wolfe, personal communications, August 8, 1983, and November 15, 1984). Total MR/DD Regional Resource Center Data for FY 1969–72 are from Braddock (1973, p. 46). Early Childhood data for FY 1969–84 were obtained from the OSE Division of Innovation and Development (R. Champion, personal communication, August 12, 1983); and FY 1985 figures were from Wolfe (personal communication, November 15, 1984). Regional Resource Center and Early Childhood MR/DD estimated expenditures were computed using the State Grant Program's annual mental retardation child count pupil participation rates. The expenditure data for the total Severely Handicapped Projects Program were obtained from the program office (P. Thompson, personal communication, August 19, 1983). Thompson estimated that 70% of total program spending annually since FY 1977 has been allocated for MR/DD–related activities. Prior to the funding of the first Severely Handicapped Projects in FY 1976, OSE supported Area Learning Resource Centers and Instructional Materials Centers under this section. Estimated MR/DD support at these centers was predicated on nationwide State Grant Program child count data applied to total program expenditures. FY 1985 appropriations were provided by Wolfe (personal communication, November 15, 1984).

the total Vocational Education State Grant Program (see Figure 15) and in services to handicapped persons (see Figure 16). Total state grant obligations, in FY 1965, were $168.6 million. Excluding a spending freeze in FY 1968, and a slight drop in FY 1969, total state grant spending advanced steadily year-to-year until FY 1976, when it dropped from $428.1 million to $422.6 million. The average rate of growth between FY 1970 and FY 1976 was 5.6% per year.

Obligations dropped by 4%, however, between FY 1977 and FY 1979. They resumed a strong upward direction in FY 1980–81, growing by 30% over the FY 1979 level to $559.8 million in FY 1981. Spending plunged

7.6% in FY 1982 after the enactment of OBRA. Since FY 1982, allocations have increased modestly, reaching a new high of $566.7 million in FY 1985.

During FY 1965–75, vocational education spending for services to all handicapped persons followed patterns identical to that for services to children and youth with mental retardation. In FY 1976, however, only 33% of all handicapped children served in the program were identified as mentally retarded, as opposed to 50% in FY 1970. The large drop in spending for services to children with mental retardation in FY 1976 is mainly attributable to the use of the new and smaller statistic. Figure 16 illustrates trends in allocations for

Severely Handicapped Projects: Total funding	Severely Handicapped Projects: Estimated MR funding	Deaf-Blind Centers: Total funding	Deaf-Blind Centers: MR funding	Instructional Media: Total funding	Instructional Media: Estimated MR funding
$1,625	$715				
$1,906	$838				
$2,956	$1,300				
$3,407	$1,260				
$4,001	$1,560	$2,000	$1,000		
$4,057	$1,338	$4,500	$2,250		
$4,253	$1,318	$7,500	$3,750		
$5,300	$1,493	$10,000	$5,000		
NA	$1,154	$14,055	$7,027		
NA	$1,154	$12,000	$6,000		
$3,250	$815	$16,000	$8,000	$19,000	500
$3,250	$2,275	$16,000	$8,000	$19,000	$500
$3,250	$2,275	$16,000	$8,000	$19,000	$500
$5,000	$3,500	$16,000	$8,000	$19,000	$500
$5,000	$3,500	$16,000	$8,000	$19,000	$500
$2,880	$2,016	$16,000	$8,000	$17,000	$410
$2,880	$2,016	$15,360	$7,680	$12,000	$410
$2,880	$2,016	$15,360	$7,680	$12,000	$410
$4,000	$2,800	$15,000	$7,500	$14,000	$800
$4,300	$3,010	$15,000	$7,500	$14,000	$1,900

Estimated spending associated with the Deaf-Blind Program is based on the conservative assumption that half of the children served are MR/DD in addition to being deaf and also blind. The OSE reported in FY 1978 House budget hearings that between 50% and 85% of "deaf-blind children had also been diagnosed as having some degree of mental retardation" (U.S. House of Representatives, 1979, p. 310). The OSE Budget Office provided total Deaf-Blind expenditures for FY 1973–85 (B. Wolfe, personal communications, August 19, 1983, and November 15, 1984); FY 1970–72 data are from Braddock (1973).

The Instructional Media Program, Part F, primarily supports activities in deafness. However, there is evidence of MR/DD media and curricular projects being funded since FY 1977. MR/DD data for FY 1976–85 reflect funding for the Vanderbilt University Curricular Center. Funding in FY 1984 supported four projects designed to enhance teaching aids for mildly and moderately handicapped students in secondary school. Funding in FY 1985 supported a continuation of the FY 1984 projects to teach mildly and moderately mentally handicapped students social skills for making the transition from school to the workplace. Data were provided by the OSE (J. Johnson, personal communication, November 20, 1984).

services to all handicapped individuals served in the Vocational Education Program.

Impact Aid

PL 81-874: Special Education/Indian Special Education In 1951, PL 81-874 and PL 81-815 authorized the first programs of federal aid to local school districts "impacted" negatively by the presence of federal installations. To be eligible for aid currently, the district must have at least 400 students, or 3% of their enrollment, from federally connected families. The Education Amendments of 1974, PL 93-380, authorized local educa-

tion agencies to receive 150% of their basic per-pupil reimbursement if the pupil is a handicapped child and is receiving appropriate services. ESEA Amendments in 1978, PL 95-561, extended reimbursement to handicapped children placed by local schools in private schools. Table 7 presents impact aid data authorized by current impact aid legislation.

Records are available documenting reimbursements for special education students for FY 1976–85. During this time, total federal spending for all handicaps more than tripled, from $16.8 million to $64.5 million (see Figure 17). The percentage of special education spending among all impact aid reimbursements rose from 3% to 10%. Reimbursements

Table 6. Vocational Education Act as Amended: Estimated federal mental retardation spending, FY 1965–85 (dollars are in thousands)

FY	Basic state grants: Tot. fed. obligations/ allocations	Expenditures for handicapped	Estimated MR expenditures
1965	$168,607	$346	$87
1966	$241,902	$1,852	$463
1967	$265,377	$3,559	$890
1968	$265,377	$6,167	$1,542
1969	$255,377	$7,884	$1,971
1970	$307,497	$21,408	$10,704
1971	$321,699	$33,872	$16,934
1972	$383,766	$37,900	$18,950
1973	$383,843	$43,235	$21,618
1974	$412,508	$42,304	$21,152
1975	$428,139	$48,224	$24,112
1976	$422,629	$48,563	$16,025
1977	$447,515	$46,046	$15,195
1978	$413,303	$44,769	$14,774
1979	$430,671	$53,140	$17,536
1980	$473,397	$63,063	$20,800
1981	$559,833	$68,448	$22,587
1982	$517,413	$70,989	$23,426
1983	$544,805	$70,824	$23,372
1984	$557,962	$72,535	$23,937
1985	$566,688	$73,669	$24,311

Source: Data for FY 1965–73 are from Braddock (1973, pp. 63–64). Estimated MR/DD obligations for FY 1974–75 are from Office of Mental Retardation Coordination (OMRC, 1973, 1974). Data for FY 1976–85 are based on administrative records of the Adult, Vocational, and Technical Education Bureau, U.S. Department of Education, (K. Chauvin, personal communication, July 14, 1983; A. Kibler, personal communication, December 3, 1984).

The FY 1965–69 data are based on a bureau program audit in 1972, which disclosed that 25% of services to, and thus of costs for, "special needs" students were for persons with mental retardation. The "special needs" category included disadvantaged and handicapped students at that time. Data for FY 1970–75 are bureau estimates based on program audits that determined that about 50% of all youth served under the 10% earmark in force for handicapped expenditures at that time were for persons with mental retardation. MR/DD data estimates for FY 1976–84 are based on an audit reported by the "Secretary's Report on Vocational Education" (U.S. Department of Education, 1982). This audit stated that only 33% of total handicapped expenditures were deployed for students with mental retardation.

Estimates on total handicapped youth served for FY 1976–79 were collected from the field by bureau staff; data for FY 1980–82 were gathered by the National Center for Education Statistics. Estimates for FY 1983–85 were extrapolated from the average of the mental retardation utilization rates for the previous 4 years (13%); these were applied to total state grant spending for FY 1976–79. One-third of these earmarked funds are estimated to be mental retarda-

tion funds, based on the secretary's 1982 report. No excess cost factor for educating youth with mental retardation has been used in the computations.

for children with mental retardation more than doubled, from $4.2 million to $9.7 million during the same period. The overall gain, however, conceals the decline in reimbursements during FY 1981–83. On an adjusted basis (see Figure 18), mental retardation reimbursements, which peaked in FY 1980, fell below the FY 1976 level in FY 1982–83, and recovered slightly in FY 1985; thus they ended up only 17% higher in real economic terms in FY 1985 than when reimbursements began in FY 1976. It should be stressed that growth in reimbursements generated by special education students occurred against a background of major cutbacks in funding for the entire Impact Aid Program. Total spending increased from $558.7 million in FY 1976, to $662.8 million in FY 1980. It then plummeted by 36% to $424.1 million in FY 1982. The FY 1985 appropriation was $643 million, slightly below unadjusted spending levels in FY 1979–80, but substantially above the FY 1983–84 level (see Table 7).

VOCATIONAL REHABILITATION SERVICES

PL 93-112 as Amended, Title I: State Grants The Vocational Rehabilitation Program is the nation's oldest state-federal assistance program authorizing the provision of services to disabled individuals. It began with the enactment of the Smith-Fess Act, the National Civilian Vocational Rehabilitation Act of 1920. Smith-Fess operated for only 4 years, however, and as a *reimbursement* program. Funds were provided on the basis of an equivalent 50% state-federal match. Services provided included training, guidance, placement, and prosthetic appliances. Mentally handicapped persons were not eligible for such services. In 1930, and again in 1932, amendments extended the act and authorized $1 million for expenditure.

In 1935, the act was incorporated into Title

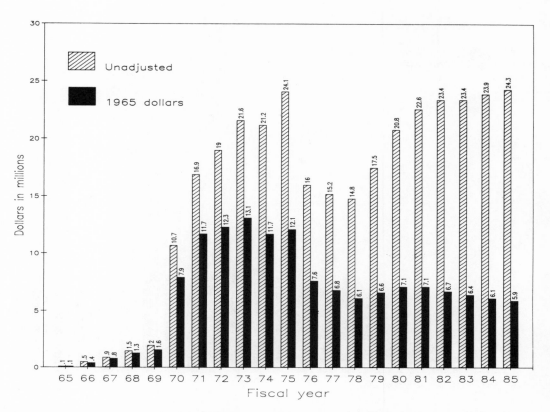

Figure 14. Estimated spending for Vocational Education State Grant services to youths with mental retardation: FY 1965–85.

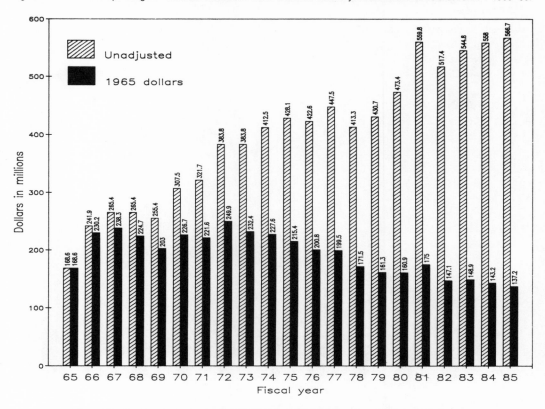

Figure 15. Total spending for the Vocational Education Act State Grant Program: FY 1965–85.

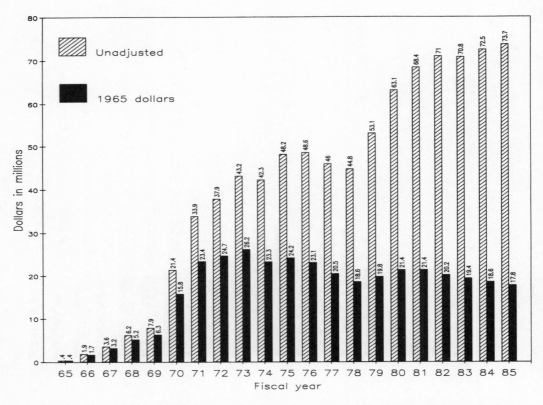

Figure 16. Spending for services to handicapped youth under the Vocational Education Act State Grant Program: FY 1965–85.

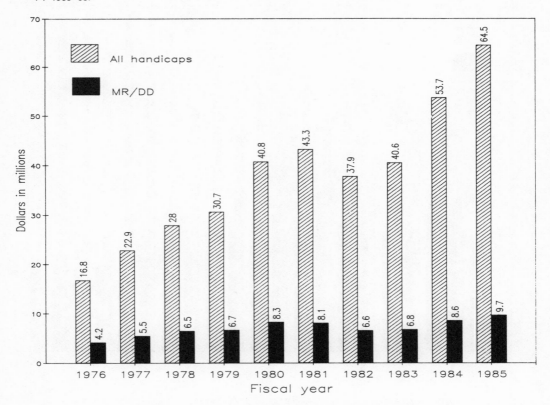

Figure 17. Impact aid funding for special education: FY 1976–85.

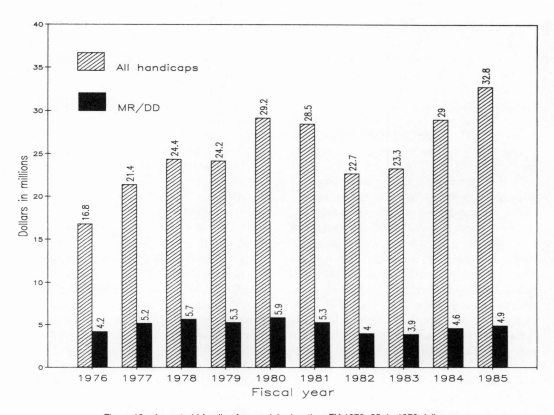

Figure 18. Impact aid funding for special education: FY 1976–85, in 1976 dollars.

Table 7. PL 81-874 as Amended: Estimated impact aid spending for students with mental retardation, FY 1976–85 (dollars are thousands)

FY	Total impact aid funds	Special education funds	% Special education	% MR in special education	Estimated MR funds
1976	$558,715	$16,792	3.00%	25.07%	$4,210
1977	$619,119	$22,851	3.70%	24.05%	$5,496
1978	$637,178	$28,000	4.40%	23.15%	$6,482
1979	$660,137	$30,702	4.70%	21.76%	$6,681
1980	$662,766	$40,830	6.20%	20.22%	$8,256
1981	$615,336	$43,341	7.00%	18.63%	$8,074
1982	$424,095	$37,897	8.90%	17.50%	$6,629
1983	$435,000	$40,591	9.20%	16.73%	$6,791
1984	$535,000	$53,697	10.03%	15.95%	$8,564
1985	$643,000	$64,493	10.03%	14.99%	$9,666

Source: Accounting records for PL 81-974 were supplied by the Impact Aid Program Office, U.S. Department of Education (C. Dexter, personal communications, December 14, 1983, January 9, 1984; and November 20, 1984). To determine estimated mental retardation expenditures, mental retardation child count percentages for PL 94-142 were applied to total annual expenditures for special education.

V of the landmark Social Security Act. The Vocational Rehabilitation Program was also made permanent, and annual appropriations were doubled to $2 million. In 1939, the authorization for such appropriations was again increased—to $3.5 million.

The Vocational Rehabilitation Amendments of 1943, the Barden-LaFollete Act, authorized the provision of services to mentally handicapped persons. (Also, medical services were authorized for physical restoration of disabled persons, as were client living expenses and travel costs.) Ten years later, reimbursement was finally abandoned and funding was converted to grants and contracts. In FY 1953, appropriations were $22.25 million. The following year, the Vocational Rehabilitation Act Amendments of 1954 linked the rehabilitation program with the Social Security Disability Insurance Trust Fund. The Vocational Rehabilitation Program was also cast in three components: 1) Basic State Grant Support, 2) Extension and Improvement, and 3) Special Projects.

The Rehabilitation Act of 1973, PL 93-112, revised, expanded, and reauthorized the Vocational Rehabilitation Program. The act was notable in its inclusion of civil rights provisions prohibiting discrimination by organizations receiving federal financial assistance and in the emphasis placed on rehabilitation of severely handicapped clients. This emphasis was restated and strengthened in the Rehabilitation, Comprehensive Services, and Developmental Disabilities Amendments of 1978 (PL 95-602). The 1978 amendments established a grant authority for supporting Independent Living Services for severely disabled persons. PL 93-112 also required for the first time an "Individual, Written Rehabilitation Plan" (IWRP), analogous to the Individualized Education Program (IEP) called for in PL 94-142.

The federal-state basic grant program operates on a 90–10 percentage matching basis and is authorized by Title I, Section 110 of the 1973 act. As shown in Table 8, the proportion of clients rehabilitated who were mentally retarded increased steadily almost without exception for 30 years—FY 1945–74. The percentage of clients with mental retardation among the total pool of persons rehabilitated reached 12.5% in FY 1971, and then began to level off.

As previously stated, vocational rehabilitation services to individuals with mental retardation were initially authorized in 1943. Funds were first expended for this purpose in FY 1945, when 106 clients with mental retardation were rehabilitated. The total number of clients rehabilitated rose annually between FY 1945 and FY 1951, except in FY 1946, and from FY 1954 to FY 1974 (see Figure 19). Total clients rehabilitated reached a peak in FY 1974 at 332,048 rehabilitants nationally, but then declined in FY 1975 to slightly less than the FY 1972 level. Declines in FY 1979–83 reflected the legislative emphasis placed on providing services to severely disabled clients. Following a decline in the number of rehabilitants in FY 1983, matching the FY 1968 level, rehabilitants were projected to rise slightly in FY 1984 and FY 1985 based on increased appropriations both years.

The rehabilitation of clients with mental retardation has followed essentially similar patterns. Numbers of clients with mental retardation rehabilitated rose annually in FY 1945–49, then flattened out for FY 1950–55 at about 1% of the total rehabilitation caseload. After the Fogarty Committee's hearings in February, 1955, the trend resumed its upward path for 16 consecutive years, FY 1956–71, rising to 12.5% of the program's total caseload. The number of persons with mental retardation who were rehabilitated dropped slightly in FY 1972, but reached a 40-year peak in FY 1974 when 41,935 persons with mental retardation, or 12.6% of the total caseload, were reported rehabilitated. The annual number of rehabilitants with mental retardation in 1975–77 declined; and from FY 1978 to FY 1984, the numbers paralleled the program's global characteristics. A slight increase was projected for FY 1984 and FY 1985, based on increases in the total State Grant Program's available appropriations. Figure 20 graphically depicts the annual number of clients with mental retarda-

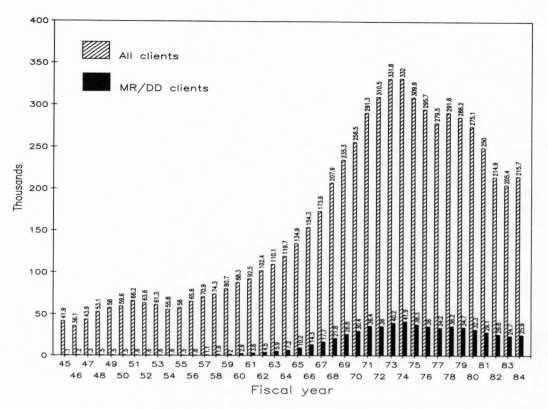

Figure 19. Number of clients rehabilitated under the state-federal Vocational Rehabilitation Program: FY 1945–84.

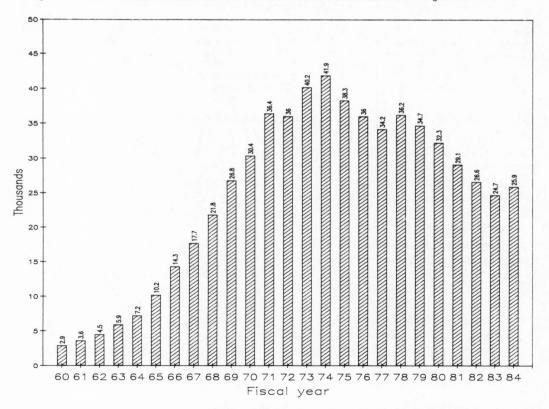

Figure 20. Number of clients with mental retardation rehabilitated under the state-federal Vocational Rehabilitation Program: FY 1960–84.

51

Table 8. Vocational Rehabilitation Act, PL 93-112 State Grant Program obligations: Mental retardation summary (dollars are in thousands)

FY	Total $	Clients rehabilitated	MR rehabilitants	% MR	Estimated MR $	Severity of MR clients (%)		
						Mild	Moderate	Severe
1945	$8,000	41,925	106	0.25%	$24			
1946	$8,258	36,106	175	0.48%	$41			
1947	$11,747	43,880	299	0.68%	$82			
1948	$18,000	53,131	479	0.90%	$162			
1949	$18,000	58,020	539	0.93%	$162			
1950	$20,500	59,597	493	0.83%	$164			
1951	$20,600	66,193	592	0.89%	$185			
1952	$21,500	63,632	615	0.97%	$215			
1953	$22,250	61,308	573	0.93%	$200			
1954	$23,000	55,825	561	1.00%	$230			
1955	$23,812	57,981	531	0.92%	$214			
1956	$28,830	65,640	756	1.15%	$332			
1957	$33,648	70,940	1,094	1.54%	$519			
1958	$39,365	74,317	1,578	2.12%	$836			
1959	$43,932	80,739	2,016	2.50%	$1,097			
1960	$48,144	88,275	2,937	3.33%	$1,602			
1961	$53,898	92,501	3,562	3.85%	$2,075			
1962	$60,986	102,377	4,458	4.35%	$2,656			
1963	$69,325	110,136	5,909	5.37%	$3,719			
1964	$82,195	119,708	7,206	6.02%	$4,948			

Source: Estimated annual mental retardation obligations were ascertained by multiplying the annual percentage of retarded clients with mental retardation rehabilitated times the total financial obligations expended under the State Grant Program. The implicit assumption is that the cost of rehabilitating the client with mental retardation is, on the average, approximately equivalent to the average cost of rehabilitating the typical handicapped client. The Office of the Commissioner of the Rehabilitation Services Administration (RSA), U.S. Department of Education (L. Mars, personal communication, July 22, 1984) indicated that this assumption is reasonable, although it may underestimate the cost since there is some indication that clients with mental retardation are about 10% more expensive to rehabilitate than average clients.

tion who were reported rehabilitated under the State-Federal Vocational Rehabilitation Program since FY 1960. It should be noted that the annual percentage of clients with mental retardation rehabilitated has remained stable since FY 1969 at between 11% and 12% of the total caseload.

Federal spending for rehabilitation state grants has expanded dramatically over the past 40 years, reflecting a rapidly growing caseload and the increasing cost of providing services. Excluding both FY 1949 and 1980, when funding was frozen at the previous year's level, expenditures grew on an unadjusted basis every year between FY 1945 and FY 1985. There were particularly large increases in funding in the FY 1956–71 period. On an unadjusted annual basis, total program

funding growth averaged 13% between FY 1956 and FY 1963, and 29% per year during FY 1963–71. Since FY 1971, the unadjusted rate of growth has moderated substantially, averaging 5.5% growth per year. Figure 21 and Figure 22 display total state grant funding trends over the 40-year period in constant and in unadjusted terms.

Estimating MR/DD expenditures under the State Grant Program involved an assumption that the rehabilitation of persons with mental retardation was no more expensive than rehabilitation of the program's typical client. This probably somewhat underestimates actual costs since clients with mental retardation may often require extended counseling, trial work, and follow-along assistance to successfully complete the rehabilitation experience.

Table 8.   *(continued)*

FY	Total $	Clients rehabilitated	MR rehabilitants	% MR	Estimated MR $	Severity of MR clients (%)		
						Mild	Moderate	Severe
1965	$94,317	134,859	10,248	7.60%	$7,167			
1966	$144,629	154,279	14,293	9.26%	$13,399			
1967	$225,268	173,594	17,724	10.21%	$23,000			
1968	$282,337	207,918	21,775	10.47%	$29,569			
1969	$340,858	235,257	26,762	11.38%	$38,775			
1970	$435,999	256,544	30,356	11.83%	$51,590			
1971	$501,997	291,272	36,409	12.50%	$62,750			
1972	$560,000	310,458	36,043	11.61%	$65,014	65%	28%	7%
1973	$589,000	331,768	40,159	12.10%	$71,296	66%	26%	8%
1974	$650,000	332,048	41,935	12.63%	$82,090	64%	28%	8%
1975	$680,000	309,948	38,338	12.37%	$84,110	60%	30%	10%
1976	$720,309	295,693	36,000	12.17%	$87,696	57%	33%	10%
1977	$740,309	279,514	34,180	12.23%	$90,528	58%	32%	10%
1978	$760,472	291,569	36,203	12.42%	$94,425	56%	34%	10%
1979	$817,484	286,172	34,651	12.11%	$98,985	56%	34%	10%
1980	$817,484	275,064	32,265	11.73%	$95,891	55%	35%	10%
1981	$854,259	249,982	29,075	11.63%	$99,357	55%	35%	10%
1982	$863,039	214,871	26,623	12.39%	$106,932			
1983	$943,899	205,419	24,650	12.00%	$113,267			
1984	$1,037,800	215,691	25,883	12.00%	$124,536			
1985	$1,117,500			12.00%	$134,100			

The number of all clients rehabilitated, and the number of clients with mental retardation rehabilitated were obtained from several sources. Data for FY 1945–69 were obtained from *Mental Retardation Sourcebook* (Office of Mental Retardation Coordination [OMRC], September, 1972, p. 120). Subsequent client data were obtained from the Office of the RSA Commissioner (L. Mars personal communication, October 25, 1984). Historical financial data for total state grant appropriations were obtained from the U.S. Senate Appropriations Subcommittee on Labor, Health, Human Services, and Education hearings records for FY 1945–54. Braddock (1973, p. 96) supplied expenditure data for FY 1955–72. The FY 1973–85 fiscal data were provided by the RSA Commissioner's Office (personal communication, October 25, 1984) and by the RSA Budget Office (G. White, personal communication, November 15, 1984).

Figure 23 depicts estimated annual mental retardation expenditures based on straightforward multiplication of the annual percentage of clients with mental retardation rehabilitated times total annual program obligations.

Inspection of the data underlying Figure 23 reveals annual increases in unadjusted mental retardation funding for FY 1956–85. In real economic terms, the growth pattern is also consistently upward through FY 1974. After FY 1974, the plateau in the percentage of clients with mental retardation rehabilitated combines with a regression in real state grant appropriations to produce declining expenditure figures, until a recent slight resurgence in FY 1983–85. In FY 1985, real dollar mental retardation rehabilitation expenditures were

down 25% from the FY 1974 level. State rehabilitation agencies, however, reported a steady increase in the number of clients with moderate and severe mental retardation they rehabilitated during the FY 1974–81 period.

Real economic growth in the overall Vocational Rehabilitation State Grant Program came to an abrupt halt in FY 1972, and it has been declining since then, until a slight resurgence in FY 1983–85. This decline in resources for the total program has had a significant and negative impact on services to individuals with mental retardation.

Vocational Rehabilitation Act: Facility Improvement (Sec. 13) and Extension and Improvement (Sec. 3)   Section 13, now ter-

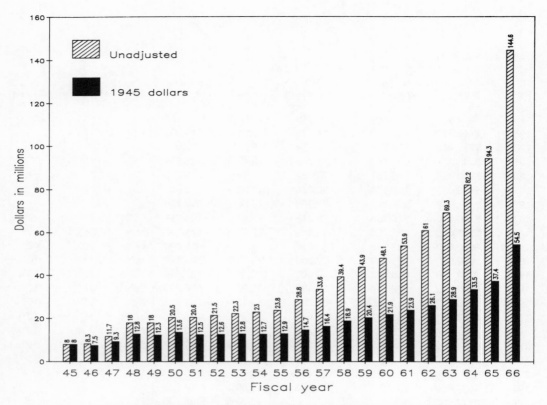

Figure 21.   Federal expenditures for the Vocational Rehabilitation State Grant Program: FY 1945–66.

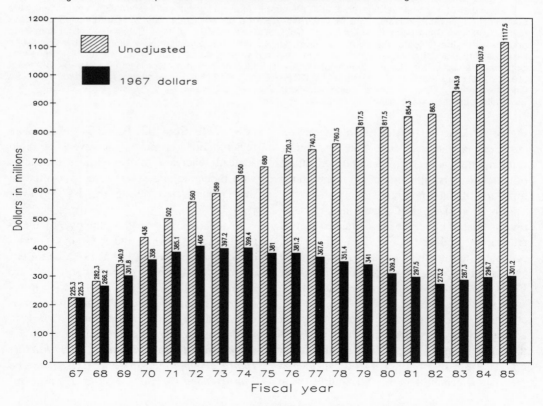

Figure 22.   Federal expenditures for the Vocational Rehabilitation State Grant Program: FY 1967–85.

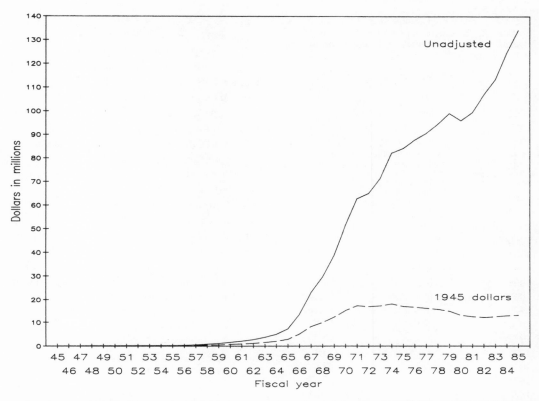

Figure 23.   Estimated mental retardation expenditures incurred under the Vocational Rehabilitation State Grant Program: FY 1945–85.

minated, was authorized by PL 89-333, the Vocational Rehabilitation Amendments of 1966, and was funded during FY 1966–79. A variety of Section 13 MR/DD projects were funded primarily in the 1970s. During FY 1972, for example, RSA reported that 197 mental retardation projects were funded. These included technical assistance to sheltered workshops, consultation on workflow, safety engineering, contract procurement, and vocational evaluation and adjustment. Projects also provided staff training and services.

Extension and Improvement Project Grants, also now terminated, were initiated during the early developmental period of the Vocational Rehabilitation Program's services to persons with mental retardation. The projects were authorized by Section 3 of PL 83-565, the Rehabilitation Amendments of 1954. They were also termed ''Innovation'' grants. The purpose of these projects was to encourage the states to develop new programs and to extend

their services to disability groups and geographical areas previously unserved or poorly served. Services to persons with mental retardation fit this category between FY 1955 and FY 1971. A total of 89 mental retardation projects were funded between FY 1955 and FY 1968. (See Table 9 for expenditure trends under Sections 3 and 13.)

PUBLIC HEALTH SERVICES

The public health services subcategory includes the following seven major health services program elements: Title XIX ICF/MR services, Title XIX Noninstitutional Medicaid, Medicare, Maternal and Child Health Services, Crippled Children's Services, Lead Based Paint Poisoning Prevention, and Civilian Health and Medical Program of the Uniformed Services (CHAMPUS). Combined FY 1985 spending for these programs constituted

Table 9.   Vocational Rehabilitation Act as Amended Section 3: Extension and Improvement Projects; Section 13: Facility Improvement Grants (dollars are in thousands)

FY	Sec. 3 funds	Sec. 13 funds
1955	$7	
1956	$89	
1957	$102	
1958	$134	
1959	$218	
1960	$203	
1961	$211	
1962	$76	
1963	$87	
1964	$186	
1965	$160	
1966	$154	$122
1967	$95	$612
1968	$142	$1,017
1969	$127	$1,140
1970	$223	$1,168
1971	$28	$1,413
1972	$0	$3,748
1973	$0	$3,150
1974	$0	$2,530
1975	$0	$2,139
1976	$0	$300
1977	$0	$314
1978	$0	$312
1979	$0	$312
1980	$0	$0
1981	$0	$0
1982	$0	$0
1983	$0	$0
1984	$0	$0
1985	$0	$0

Source: Data for Section 13 for FY 1966–71 are from Braddock (1973, p. 96). Data for FY 1972–74 are from FY 1974 House Appropriations Hearings "Supplementary Data" (Office of Mental Retardation Coordination [OMRC], 1973, p. 65); data for FY 1974–76 are from "House Hearings" (OHI, 1976, p. 67); data for FY 1977–79 are from House hearings on the FY 1981 budget (U.S. House of Representatives [House], 1980, p. 643). All of these figures were based on RSA staff inspection of Section 13 grant records.

Section 3 was funded between FY 1955 and FY 1971. Data are from Braddock (1973, p. 96). Braddock reviewed Section 3 project grant titles and descriptions for all Section 3 projects funded between FY 1955 and FY 1968. Data for FY 1969–71 were obtained from records inspected by the RSA Division of the Project Grants Administration (Braddock, 1973).

82% of all federal MR/DD services expenditures, and about half of all federal government MR/DD expenditures. The pie chart in Figure 24 depicts the composition of the seven major elements of the federal public health services MR/DD mission. In addition, there are two other smaller programs in this category that operated for several years in the 1960s—Hospital Staff Development and State Mental Retardation Planning.

Public health programs are administered by two federal departments. Most of the programs are in the Public Health Service of the Department of Health and Human Services. One program, CHAMPUS, is in the Department of Defense.

Social Security Act, Title XIX: ICF/MR Program   The ICF/MR Program grew out of the 1965 Amendments to the Social Security Act, PL 89-97, which established a new Title XIX authorizing grants-in-aid to states for the operation of medical assistance programs. Title XIX expanded the Kerr-Mills Program of medical aid for needy, aged, blind, disabled, and dependent persons. Medicaid was targeted specifically at two eligible populations: those receiving public assistance, who were designated "categorically needy"; and persons above the poverty level who, at the discretion of the state, could be designated "medically needy."

The ICF/MR Program was launched with the enactment of PL 92-223, the Social Security Amendments of 1971. That legislation authorized "Intermediate Care Facility" (ICF) services to be reimbursed under Medicaid instead of under Title XI of the Social Security Act. ICF services were defined as services in institutional settings, which did not require the high degree of care and treatment called for in a hospital or skilled nursing facility. For MR/DD persons, however, the key provision of the act was the authorization of public institutions to receive Title XIX reimbursements. To receive these funds, states had to ensure that residents were receiving "active treatment."

In the next decade, the ICF/MR Program grew to become the single largest source of

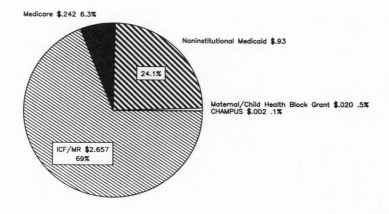

Total: $3.851 Billion

Figure 24.   Estimated federal spending for MR/DD public health services by program: FY 1985. (Dollars are in billions.)

federal funds for the operation of state institutions, and an important source of funds for community services operations including "15-bed or less" facilities. In 1981, the Omnibus Budget Reconciliation Act authorized waivers permitting states to provide alternative community-based home care and related services, provided that states could meet a rigorous cost test that required such services to be demonstrably cheaper than institutional care. As of January, 1985, 45 states had been granted waivers by the Health Care Financing Administration (National Association of State Mental Retardation Program Directors [National Association] 1985).

In FY 1984, 75% of the total of $2.572 billion in federal ICF/MR reimbursements went to the states for institutional operations. The remaining 25% provided assistance for publicly and privately operated community-based services. The growth of the program has been explosive. Federal funding advanced in unadjusted terms from $92.2 million in FY 1973 to $2.657 billion in FY 1985 (see Table 10). Even on an adjusted basis, growth averaged 24% per year between FY 1973 and FY 1985. As shown in Figure 25, however, program growth has slowed considerably since FY 1982 and the implementation of Medicaid cost-containment sanctions. During FY 1982–85, real growth averaged only 1.4% annually.

On an adjusted basis, ICF/MR reimbursements were projected to fall slightly in FY 1985 for the first time.

During its period of accelerated growth, FY 1972–81, the ICF/MR Program was the fastest growing medical assistance program supported by Title XIX (Medicaid). While federal Medicaid funding advanced from $3.527 billion in 1972 to $22.116 billion in FY 1985 (Figure 26), the percentage of ICF/MR reimbursements of the total program increased from 1% to 12% (see Figure 27); moreover, that 12% of total Medicaid payments devoted to ICF/MR services is being spent on only .7% of the total Medicaid caseload of about 23 million persons. As shown in Figure 28, the number of ICF/MR recipients served increased rapidly from 12,200 in FY 1972, to a peak of 151,200 in FY 1981.

In FY 1984, federal ICF/MR reimbursements were $18,231 per year for each of the 141,100 recipients. This was an average federal ICF/MR per diem payment of $49.95 per day in both institutional and community settings combined. In FY 1984, ICF/MR reimbursements constituted 45% of total state-federal spending for institutional operations in the United States.

Social Security Act, Title XIX: Noninstitutional Medicaid   The state of New York was the first to enact a public welfare statute spe-

Table 10. History of ICF/MR reimbursements: FY 1972–84 (dollars are in thousands)

FY	Total Title XIX federal funding	ICF/MR reimbursements (federal share)	% ICF/MR of total (federal share)	Number of ICF/MR recipients	Total Medicaid recipients
1972(e)[a]	$3,527,467	$36,872	1.05%	12,188	18,311,978
1973	$4,838,260	$92,181	1.91%	30,472	19,998,566
1974	$5,590,413	$113,835	2.04%	40,008	22,008,607
1975	$6,873,890	$195,174	2.84%	55,033	22,413,309
1976	$7,913,889	$336,904	4.26%	85,633	24,666,253
1977	$9,114,477	$615,337	6.75%	100,823	22,929,873
1978	$10,066,544	$817,393	8.12%	100,496	22,206,577
1979	$11,458,642	$1,080,462	9.43%	115,168	21,536,715
1980	$13,291,174	$1,479,285	11.13%	125,328	21,710,516
1981	$15,739,472	$1,833,670	11.65%	151,235	21,979,638
1982	$16,743,303	$2,170,314	12.96%	148,728	21,936,446
1983	$17,751,945	$2,395,178	13.49%	151,036	21,493,000
1984	$19,884,000	$2,572,336	12.94%	141,079	22,487,000

Source: All data for FY 1973–76, and recipient data for FY 1973–80, were provided by the Health Care Financing Administration (HCFA), Office of Financial and Actuarial Analysis, Medicaid Statistics Branch (R. Beisel, personal communication, February 1983); recipient figures for FY 1981–84 were also provided by that office (T. Parker, personal communication, March 11, 1986). Mental retardation fiscal data for FY 1977–84 are from the analysis of state ICF/MR data gathered by Braddock, Hemp, and Howes (1984).

MR/DD fiscal and client data for FY 1972 are the author's estimates. According to the FY 1973 House appropriations hearings record, 6 months of federal ICF/MR reimbursements were apparently expended in FY 1972. (HCFA is unable to confirm this.) However, the FY 1973 hearings record (OMRC, 1974) indicates that 28 states had filed annual Medicaid state plans by April 1, 1972. They apparently took advantage of the fact that PL 92-223 authorized ICF/MR reimbursements commencing January 1, 1972. The FY 1972 figure entered in the table above assumes that the FY 1972 figure would be less than 50% of the FY 1973 figure provided by HCFA ($92,181), since the program only operated for 6 months in FY 1972, and several new states may have joined the program in FY 1973. It has been arbitrarily assumed that the FY 1972 reimbursements and recipients served figures might conservatively be pegged at 40% of the FY 1973 figures.

[a]Estimated.

cifically designed to provide medical care for persons not destitute, but unable to afford medical services. The Federal Emergency Relief Act of 1933 (FERA) was the initial federal legislative statute in this area enacted by Congress. FERA ''Rules and Regulations'' authorized ''medicine, medical supplies, and medical attendants in the home, but the cost of hospitalization is excluded'' (Falk & Geddes, 1941).

The Social Security Act of 1935 explicitly prohibited federal funds from being used for medical care. Some states were able to provide medical care and hospitalization from state and local funds. Falk and Geddes (1941) stated that in January–August, 1940, 9 states provided some payments for medical care and hospitalization in their Old Age Assistance Program; 9 did so under their Aid to Dependent Children Program; and 16 authorized medical care in their Aid to the Blind Program. In addition, some additional states may have included small cash sums for medical care in their payments to needy individuals.

As noted in the immediately preceding section, PL 89-97 authorized the Medicaid medical assistance program in 1965. This legislation broke radically with the early tradition of the Social Security Act, which had forbade federal support for such assistance. Under this program, states must provide ''categorically needy'' public assistance recipients (and may provide ''medically needy'' persons) with inpatient and outpatient hospital services, other laboratory and X ray services, skilled nursing home services, home health services, family

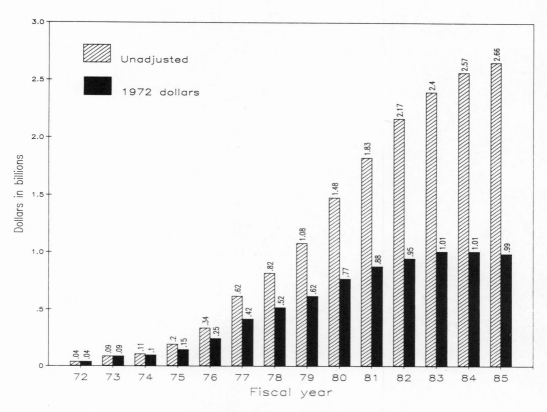

Figure 25.   Federal ICF/MR reimbursements: FY 1972–85.

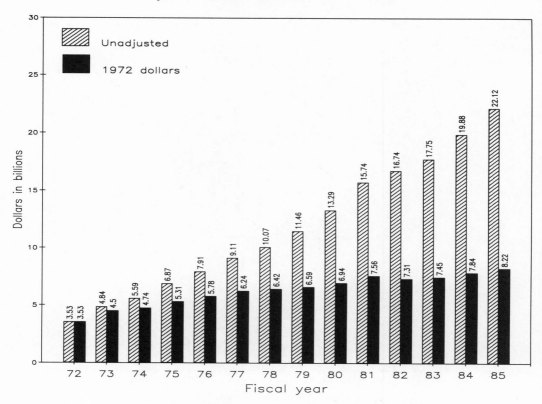

Figure 26.   The growth of federal Medicaid (Title XIX) funds: FY 1972–85.

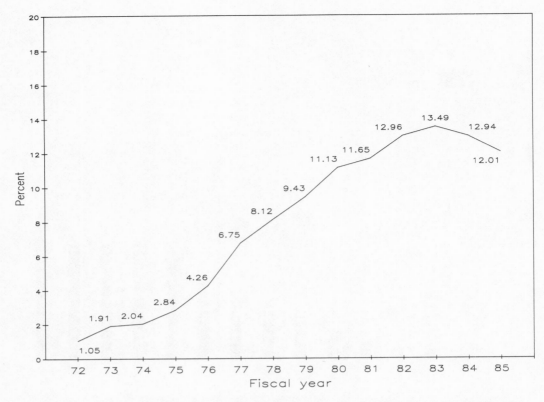

Figure 27.   The growth of federal ICF/MR reimbursements as a percentage of total Medicaid costs: FY 1972–85.

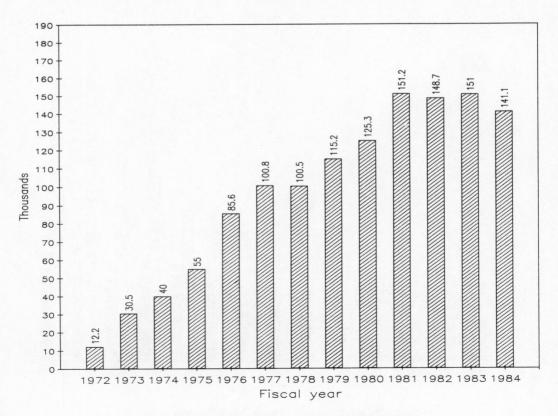

Figure 28.   Number of residents in ICF/MR settings: FY 1972–84.

planning services, and physician services. The federal government reimburses states for between 50% and 77% of the total approved cost of providing services to eligible individuals.

Most individuals with mental retardation or developmental disabilities reside in community settings (including the family home), and many of these persons are eligible for and receive Medicaid assistance or "green card" services. Eligibility criteria vary from state to state, but in general, an individual is automatically categorically eligible if he or she meets stipulated poverty guidelines, or is currently receiving public assistance such as Supplemental Security Income (SSI). Many states also define a "medically needy" category, which broadens eligibility to include certain "non-poor" (those not receiving public assistance) who have significant medical bills. However, 15 states have more restrictive eligibility criteria for Medicaid than for SSI.

Noninstitutional Medicaid refers to medical payments for eligible clients who are not living in institutional settings. HCFA data are classified simply by the three broad diagnostic categories: Aged, Blind, and Disabled. The author estimated the subset of the Blind and Disabled who are mentally retarded or developmentally disabled. Table 11 presents the author's estimates of the MR/DD share of noninstitutional Medicaid reimbursements for FY 1967–85.

On an adjusted basis, federal noninstitutional Medicaid increased steadily from FY 1967 to FY 1972 (see Figure 29). Reimbursements dipped slightly in real economic terms

Table 11. Estimated federal share of noninstitutional Medicaid reimbursements for individuals with MR/DD: 1967–85 (dollars in thousands)

FY	MR/DD reimbursements	FY	MR/DD reimbursements
1967	$54,415	1977	$417,579
1968	$65,869	1978	$449,667
1969	$82,068	1979	$535,270
1970	$100,995	1980	$595,866
1971	$129,291	1981	$656,462
1972	$157,587	1982	$717,425
1973	$133,547	1983	$746,350
1974	$153,565	1984	$835,912
1975	$182,697	1985	$929,534
1976	$221,115		

Source: To determine noninstitutional Medicaid reimbursements for MR/DD persons, the following procedures were used. Data were obtained from HCFA's Statistical Reporting Tables which are taken from the HCFA Form 2082, Annual Medicaid Statistical Reports from the states (HCFA, Office of Financial and Actuarial Analysis, Medicaid Statistics Branch, personal communications, October 28, 1983, and April 5, 1984). The author's analysis was confined to the "Blind" and "Disabled" Medicaid categories; the expenditures under the "Aged" category were not included. First, the institutional services expenditures (mental hospitals, ICFs, and skilled nursing facilities [SNFs] service categories) were subtracted from the total Medicaid figure for the Blind and Disabled categories. That calculation resulted in a total noninstitutional figure for all Blind and Disabled Medicaid recipients. Then, the portion of that figure represented by MR/DD clients was estimated at 25% (the same method used to estimate the MR/DD portion of SSI recipients, as explained in the forthcoming Income Maintenance chapter of this book).

This methodology is imperfect. It overstated MR/DD participation because the 25% factor was applied to payments to "cash" and "non-cash" recipients combined, due to the fact that historical Medicaid data combined these two categories of recipients. In fact, the 25% factor applied only to the "cash" Blind and Disabled recipients (i.e., those on SSI). This overestimating flaw may be offset by the fact that this method also assumed that MR/DD Medicaid recipients were no more expensive to serve, which is very unlikely and therefore resulted in underestimating MR/DD payments. Due to the limitations of the historical Medicaid data, this was the best possible estimating method. A number of people in HCFA and in state Medicaid offices were consulted, including: R. Beisel (Office of Financial and Actuarial Analysis), S. Meskin (Chief of the Medicaid Cost Estimates Branch), M. Brown (Chief of Long-Term Care Services Branch), J. Jackson (Medicaid Eligibility Policy Office), G. Soloway (Wisconsin), G. Gesaman (Iowa), and J. Crosby (Michigan).

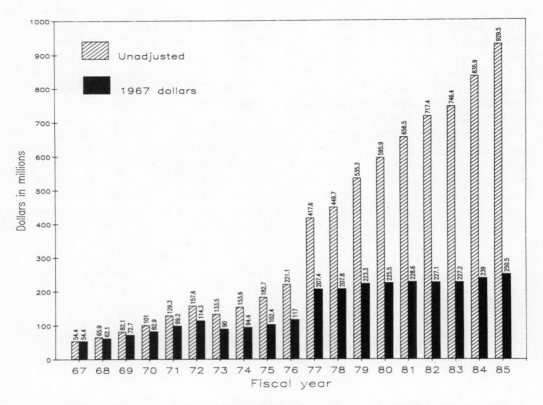

Figure 29. Estimated federal noninstitutional Medicaid reimbursements for services to persons with MR/DD: FY 1967–85.

during FY 1973–75, as the states implemented new Title XIX claims under the ICF/MR Program. Growth in reimbursements continued during FY 1976–79, but plateaued during the 1980–83 inflationary period. MR/DD projections for FY 1984–85 are derived from August, 1984, state Medicaid reports for these years, and reflect increases of 12% and 11.2%, respectively.

Social Security Act, Title XVIII: Medicare The Social Security Amendments of 1965, PL 89-97, established a program of hospital and medical insurance for the aged. The program went into effect on July 1, 1966 (except for extended care facility services which became effective on January 1, 1967). The program is authorized under Title XVIII of the Social Security Act. Under the Social Security Amendments of 1972 (PL 92-603), Medicare coverage was authorized for disabled Social Security beneficiaries after they have fulfilled

a 24-month waiting period. These amendments, authorizing Medicare coverage, affect persons with MR/DD because they are eligible for Social Security under the Adult Disabled Child (ADC) Program. Therefore, when MR/DD beneficiaries reach age 18, they continue to receive Social Security benefits. The 24-month waiting period for Medicare coverage is usually avoided by formally applying for benefits when the child is age 16.

There are two parts of the program: Hospital Insurance (Part A) and Supplementary Medical Insurance (Part B). Part A covers short-term inpatient hospitalization, related care in SNFs, and some home care. The money to pay for these services comes from Social Security taxes paid by working people, and from contributions made by their employers. Supplementary Medical Insurance (Part B), is a voluntary program which provides coverage for physician services, outpatient services, ambulance services, certain medical supplies, and durable medical equipment. It should be noted that Medicare Parts A and B cover acute, short-term hospital care, physician visits, drugs, etc. Custodial care for MR/DD beneficiaries is not ordinarily covered by Medicare except in certain cases requiring skilled nursing care.

It is important to distinguish Medicare from Medicaid. First, Medicare is an insurance program; recipients are eligible only if they have contributed to Social Security. Medicaid is a medical assistance program for needy persons, usually persons receiving public assistance. Second, Medicare is administered and funded entirely by the federal government through a trust fund. Medicaid is a federal-state grant-in-aid program subject to the general appropriations process. Overall responsibility for the administration of Medicare rests with the Secretary of the Department of Health and Human Services; specific responsibility for administration of the program was given to the Health Care Financing Administration. They determine individual eligibility, negotiate contracts, and establish regulations and standards. (For an additional discussion of the Medicaid Program, consult the two immediately preceding sections, under the Title XIX ICF/MR Program and noninstitutional Medicaid.)

As Table 12 illustrates, total funding for Parts A and B for disabled persons (excluding End Stage Renal Disease [ESRD]) jumped from $831 million in FY 1974, to $7.12 billion in FY 1984. Estimated payments to persons with mental retardation and developmental disabilities increased from $24.9 million to $213.6 million on an unadjusted basis during the same period. Projected FY 1985 funding for non-ESRD disabled beneficiaries, based on 1985 appropriations, was $8.055 billion. Of this sum, $241.65 million was estimated for persons with MR/DD, as shown in Figure 30.

On an adjusted basis, MR/DD funds grew almost every year during FY 1974–85. Real growth averaged 21% per year from FY 1974

Table 12. Estimated Medicare reimbursements for persons with MR/DD: FY 1974–85 (dollars are in thousands)

FY	Total (Parts A+B) Medicare payments to disabled, excluding ESRD	Estimated MR/DD payments
1974	$831,000	$24,930
1975	$1,198,000	$35,940
1976	$2,077,000	$62,310
1977	$2,156,000	$64,680
1978	$2,754,000	$89,144
1979	$3,234,000	$97,020
1980	$3,904,000	$117,120
1981	$4,741,000	$142,230
1982	$5,691,000	$170,730
1983	$6,320,000	$189,600
1984	$7,120,000	$213,600
1985	$8,055,000	$241,650

Source: Medicare reimbursements paid on behalf of MR/DD persons were calculated based on an unpublished utilization study by the Office of Research and Demonstrations. The 1983 study indicated that 3% of all Part A and Part B payments made in FY 1978 to disabled Social Security beneficiaries (excluding persons with End Stage Renal Disease [ESRD]) were paid to Adult Disabled Child (ADC) beneficiaries. These beneficiaries are the same individuals also receiving ADC benefits under the Social Security Disability Insurance (SSDI) Program. About 70% of ADC beneficiaries are estimated to be mentally retarded or developmentally disabled. Information about this study and the data in Table 12 were obtained from the HCFA Statistical Information Services Unit, Division of Information Analysis, Bureau of Data Management and Strategy (P. Pine, personal communication, November 22, 1983; D. Wood, personal communication, November 23, 1983).

to FY 1980, but it tapered off to 8% annually during the FY 1980–84 period.

Social Security Act, Title V, Section 503 (Maternal and Child Health Grants) and Section 504 (Crippled Children's Grants) The Maternal and Child Health (MCH) State Formula Grant Program authorized the provision of services targeted on reducing infant mortality and improving the health of mothers and children. The program has been concerned for many years with reducing the incidence of mental retardation and other handicapping conditions caused by complications associated with childbearing. The Crippled Children's

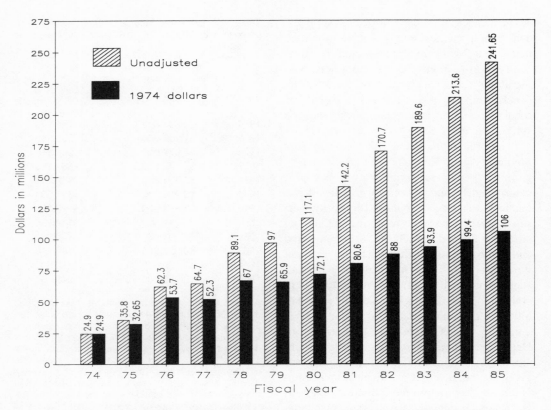

Figure 30.   Estimated federal Medicare reimbursements for services to persons with MR/DD: FY 1974–85.

(CC) Services State Grant Program seeks to provide medical and related services to handicapped children. "Crippled children" were broadly defined in the act to include children under the age of 21 with an organic disease, defect, or condition that might hinder normal growth and development.

In 1982, these two formula grant programs were combined into the Maternal and Child Health Block Grant. As individual categorical state formula grants, however, both programs have a long history and a rich tradition of service to the nation's mentally retarded and developmentally disabled children and their families.

In 1921, Congress enacted the Maternity and Infancy Act. Also known as "Sheppard-Towner," this act was the nation's first health services formula grant program. The program operated for 8 years. In 1935, the Social Security Act adopted two provisions in Title V

authorizing state grants in Maternal and Child Health and Crippled Children's Services. Annual funds authorized for expenditure were $3.8 million and $2.85 million, respectively.

As originally implemented, however, the Title V Crippled Children's Program was intended to provide services only to orthopedically handicapped children. This was clarified at the October 9–10, 1936, National Advisory Committee on Services for Crippled Children meeting:

> It was recommended that children whose chief disability is incurable blindness, deafness, or mental defect, and those having abnormalities requiring permanent custodial care should be beyond the scope of the program. (Social Security Board, 1946, p. 2)

By 1941, there were 2,291 prenatal clinics nationally; their number jumped to 2,600 in 1942. Hospital care was, however, provided in only about a dozen states, and organized home delivery nursing services were provided in only 131 counties in the United States.

In 1946, however, the Maternal and Child Health and Crippled Children's Advisory Committees met jointly, and apparently for the first time called "attention to the special needs of children with rheumatic fever, cerebral palsy, speech and hearing defects, epilepsy and chronic illness" (Social Security Board, 1946, p. 5). The advisory committees jointly recommended a "national fact-finding survey" on the "present situation with regard to the incidence and prevalence of cerebral palsy and [of] other factors affecting the care and treatment of such children" (p. 5). Medical school training programs for working with children with cerebral palsy were also encouraged. In addition, the following recommendation with specific respect to children with MR/DD was issued:

> [The Children's Bureau should] . . . ascertain the numbers and situation of cerebral palsied and other orthopedically handicapped children in institutions for the mentally deficient. (Social Security Board, 1946, p. 5)

A special report of the joint advisory committee was presented on mental health services. It recommended that the Children's Bureau hire a full-time mental health specialist, and that federal, state, and local agencies work together to establish "child guidance clinics with broadly construed mental hygiene functions" (Social Security Board, 1946, p. 15). The report also recommended that more "special hospital facilities be established in population centers to care for emotionally troubled children who could not be cared for in their own homes or in foster care" (p. 16). The 1946 report was also seminal in the area of recommending that all birth certificates include infant birth weight. Babies weighing less than 2,500 grams (5.5 pounds) required "prenatal care and pediatric consultation" (p. 10).

Amendments to the original 1935 Social Security Act increased authorization levels in 1939, 1946, and 1950. Expenditures for Maternal and Child Health Program services were $12.319 million in FY 1954; Crippled Chil-

dren's Program services were funded at a level of $11.082 million (Lesser, 1964). Hornmuth (1964) reported that in 1949, however, there was not a single child guidance clinic in the United States specializing in the provision of continuing services to children with mental retardation and their families.

Five years later, and largely due to the efforts of newly formed state Associations for Retarded Children, there were 33 clinics and 12 more were planned for 1956. Although the definition of what constituted a special clinic varied, by 1957 "75 community clinical programs for the retarded in various parts of the country could be listed . . ." (Hornmuth, 1964).

Another step forward in the provision of services to children occurred in 1954. The Children's Bureau, which administered the formula grant programs, provided a special project grant to Children's Hospital in Los Angeles to set up a diagnostic clinic for children with mental retardation. In 1955, the states of Hawaii and Washington and the District of Columbia were awarded similar clinic grants.

Congressional interest in mental retardation was expressed in February, 1955, during the House appropriations hearings on the Department of Health, Education, and Welfare (DHEW) budget for FY 1956. Chairman John Fogarty pressed DHEW officials on the need for a broad-based program of state assistance and research and development. In the FY 1957 DHEW appropriations bill, Fogarty's committee earmarked $1 million specifically for the purpose of mental retardation services through Maternal and Child Health State Grants. In FY 1962, these clinics served approximately 25,000 children with mental retardation and their families. There were 110 special clinics in FY 1962 (U.S. House of Representatives [House], 1963). Between FY 1956 and FY 1961, 484 children with phenylketonuria (PKU) were also detected and placed on special dietary supervision.

PL 88-156 (Maternal and Child Health and Mental Retardation Planning Act), incorporated several recommendations of the President's

Panel on Mental Retardation (1962). Authorization levels for the MCH and CC State Formula Grants were doubled. Maternity and Infant Care Projects also were authorized, and a special state planning grant program was adopted.

Over the next decade, 10%–20% of total funds budgeted for Sections 503 and 504 were expanded for services to MR/DD children and their families. The House Appropriations Committee hearings record for FY 1975 DHEW appropriations (OMRC, 1974) indicated that there were 166 special MCH clinics in FY 1973 operating in 48 states. Services were delivered to 75,618 children with MR/DD that year.

In 1967, PL 90-248 consolidated MCH and CC services under a single grant authorization, with funding split 50% for formula grants, 40% for project grants, and 10% for research and training. In July, 1972, the 40% share for special projects was incorporated into the state formula grant. In FY 1982, the state grants were folded into a new Maternal and Child Health Block Grant along with Lead Based Paint Poisoning Prevention Act funds, Genetic Diseases Act appropriations, and several other health services programs.

Figure 31 illustrates general trends in federal funding for MR/DD services under Section 503–504 programs (see Table 13 for dollar amounts in MR/DD obligations). The programs prospered visibly in the years following the convening of the President's Panel on Mental Retardation (1962), which issued recommendations that the programs be greatly expanded. In FY 1966, $9.9 million and $7.7 million were obligated for Section 503 and Section 504 MR/DD services, respectively. By FY 1972, however, the MR/DD resources

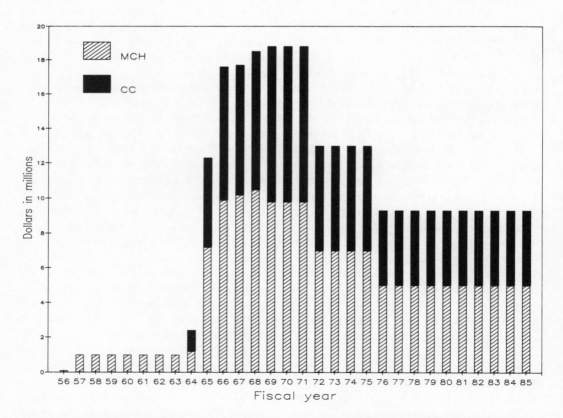

Figure 31.   Estimated federal MR/DD spending for Maternal and Child Health (MCH) and Crippled Children's (CC) services (Sections 503 and 504): FY 1956–85.

Table 13. Maternal and Child Health and Crippled Children's (Social Security Act, Sections 503 and 504) State Formula Grant MR/DD obligations: FY 1956–85 (dollars are in thousands)

FY	Section 503	Section 504	FY	Section 503	Section 504
1956	$88		1971	$9,775	$9,000
1957	$1,000		1972	$6,988	$6,002
1958	$1,000		1973	$6,988	$6,002
1959	$1,000		1974	$6,988	$6,002
1960	$1,000		1975	$6,988	$6,002
1961	$1,000		1976	$5,000	$4,321
1962	$1,000		1977	$5,000	$4,321
1963	$1,000		1978	$5,000	$4,321
1964	$1,250	$1,250	1979	$5,000	$4,321
1965	$7,152	$5,092	1980	$5,000	$4,321
1966	$9,870	$7,742	1981	$5,000	$4,321
1967	$10,205	$7,500	1982	$5,000	$4,321
1968	$10,500	$8,005	1983	$5,000	$4,321
1969	$9,775	$9,000	1984	$5,000	$4,321
1970	$9,775	$9,000	1985	$5,000	$4,321

Source: FY 1956–72 data are from Braddock (1973, p. 83). FY 1972–73 data are from OMRC (1974); FY 1974–76 data are from OHI (1975). According to Maternal and Child Health Services (MCHS) Program officials, estimated support for MR/DD services after FY 1976 continued at approximately the same utilization levels. In FY 1982, both state formula grants (Sections 503 and 504) were folded into the Maternal and Child Health Block Grant. At the author's request, agency staff inspected Block Grant expenditure reports from the states for references on mental retardation and developmental disabilities services on two occasions (R. Hornmuth, personal communications, November 29, 1983, and November 27, 1984). Evidence could not be found suggesting any change in federal support for Section 503/504 MR/DD services since FY 1976. This was the last year the agency identified a specific mental retardation expenditure in hearings before the House Appropriations Subcommittee. There was some evidence to suggest that the states have increased their own-source contributions to the operation of clinics serving children with developmental disabilities. Hornmuth (personal communications, November 29, 1983, and November 27, 1984) reported an overall increase in the number of clinics providing Section 503 services. Sections 503 and 504 supported between $4 and $6 million for informal, state-initiated training activities. (These funds are excluded from this table and appear later in the MCHS Training Program profile; see Chapter 4).

reported deployed by DHEW in congressional budget hearings fell to $6.99 million and $6 million for Sections 503 and 504, respectively. An unadjusted drop in estimated expenditures to $5 million and $4.3 million, respectively, was reported in FY 1976 budget hearings. Since there is no basis for assuming these levels have changed, the FY 1977–85 estimates merely carry forward the FY 1976 figures.

In real economic terms, the funds annually expended under these programs attributable to MR/DD services declined slightly from FY 1957 to FY 1963; increased sixfold from FY 1964 to FY 1966; leveled off in FY 1967–68; and then steadily declined during FY 1969–85. (These trends are shown in Figure 32.) Data estimating MR/DD services after FY

1972 are of poor quality, and serve only to underscore the contemporary need for a program monitoring and data collection system to gather routine information on the extent to which MR/DD services are provided under the Maternal and Child Health Services Block Grant.

Public Health Services Act, Section 314 (c) and 314 (e) The authority offered by Section 314 (c) and (e) was a historically important source of fiscal support for services development project grants in mental retardation. The authorization originally stemmed from an appropriations earmarking in FY 1962. Between FY 1947 and FY 1964, cancer, radiological health, tuberculosis, chronic illness, diseases of the aged, neurological and sensory diseases, and mental retardation were earmarked under

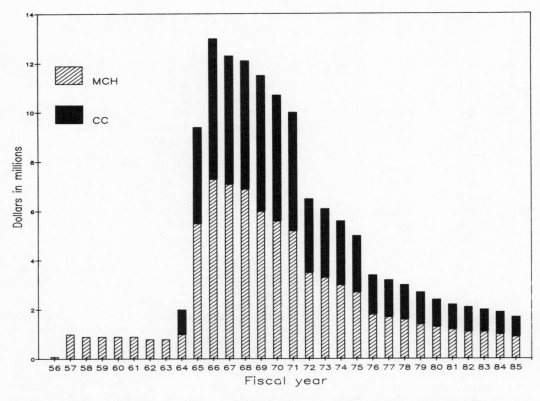

Figure 32.   Estimated federal MR/DD spending for MCH and CC services: FY 1956–85, in 1956 dollars.

Section 314 (c) of the Public Health Services Act. Then, the Comprehensive Health Planning and Public Health Service Act Amendments of 1966 reframed Section 314 (c) as Section 314 (e). The new legislation emphasized decategorization around noncategorical target populations, such as poverty, rather than by disease. By FY 1971, mental retardation support evaporated. Funding levels are presented in Table 14.

PL 91-695: Lead Based Paint Poisoning Prevention   The Lead Based Paint Poisoning Prevention Program was inaugurated in FY 1971, under PL 91-695; in FY 1982, the grant program was consolidated into the Maternal and Child Health Block Grant, administered by the Health Services Administration in the Department of Health and Human Services. Under the block grant, states acquired the leadership role for promoting and implementing lead based paint poisoning prevention ser-

vices at the local level. In a typical year, this program worked with between 50 and 60 communities, and screened between 370,000 and 440,000 children, of which between 16,000 and 26,500 were found to be lead toxic (OHI, 1976; U.S. House of Representatives, 1979,

Table 14.   Mental retardation funding under Section 314 (c) and (e) of the Public Health Service Act (dollars are in thousands)

FY	Funding
1962	$230
1963	$630
1964	$725
1965	$3,250
1966	$4,500
1967	$5,462
1968	$3,939
1969	$3,379
1970	$584

Source: Braddock (1973, p. 133).

Table 15. Lead Based Paint Poisoning Prevention Act obligations: FY 1971–85 (dollars are in thousands)

FY	Funds obligated
1971	$158
1972	$7,500
1973	$7,805
1974	$7,255
1975	$5,812
1976	$5,959
1977	$8,500
1978	$10,250
1979	$13,498
1980	$11,790
1981	$10,723
1982	$10,723
1983	$10,723
1984	$10,723
1985	$10,723

Source: Data for FY 1971–72 are from Braddock (1973, p. 89). Data for FY 1973–75 are from House hearings (OMRC, 1974, Appendix, p. 1). Data for FY 1976–77 are from 1976 House hearings (Office for Handicapped Individuals [OHI], 1975, p. 65). Data for FY 1978 are from House hearings for FY 1981 (U.S. House of Representatives [House], 1980, p. 641). Data for FY 1979–81 are from 1983 House hearings (U.S. House of Representatives [House], 1982, p. 541). Figures for FY 1982–85 assumed continuation of program spending in the states at the same level of funds expended prior to implementation of the MCH Block Grant.

1980). The DHHS Center for Disease Control indicated in FY 1983 House hearings that over the 10-year period of operation of this program, 3.7 million children were screened and 243,000 were found to be lead toxic. (Table 15 shows the funding for the program.)

PL 88-156: State Planning in Mental Retardation PL 88-156 added a new Title XVII to the Social Security Act. This program operated for 4 years, FY 1964–67. Funds obligated were $2.2 million, $2.2 million, $2.75 million, and $2.75 million, respectively (Braddock, 1973, p. 141). (Consult the preceding discussion of the Maternal and Child Health/Crippled Children's Formula Grants for background information.)

Department of Defense: Civilian Health and Medical Program of the Uniformed Services (CHAMPUS) The CHAMPUS Program for the "mentally handicapped" actually serves only individuals with MR/DD. The program pays part of the cost of residential (institutional) services and nonresidential services to members of the uniformed services, or to retirees with MR/DD dependents. Table 16 has incomplete detail for FY 1969–77 in terms of residential versus nonresidential data. Total payment levels, however, combining both categories are presented in the "Total Payments" column. (See Figure 33 for an illustration of the CHAMPUS payments in unadjusted and 1969 dollars for FY 1969–85.)

HUMAN DEVELOPMENT SERVICES

The human development services subcategory includes three major components: 1) Developmental Disabilities (DD) Act–authorized services (PL 88-164 as Amended) including State Grants, Protection and Advocacy (P&A) Grants, and Special Project Funds; 2) the Social Services Block Grant—formerly Title XX; and 3) volunteer services (the Foster Grandparent Program). Other relevant human development services programs include child welfare services, Project Head Start, and Job Training Act Services. Figure 34 illustrates the composition and volume of FY 1985 funding for MR/DD human development services. Developmental Disabilities Act funds for the operation of University Affiliated Facilities (UAFs) were considered training instead of services expenditures, and thus were omitted from Figure 34.

Developmental Disabilities Act as Amended The Developmental Disabilities Act grew out of PL 88-164, the Mental Retardation Facilities and Community Mental Health Centers Construction Act of 1963, which had embodied several of the major recommendations of the President's Panel on Mental Retardation (1962). Over the years, amendments to the act have expanded the services authorized for persons with MR/DD.

Profile The 1963 act (PL 88-164) authorized three interrelated construction programs: Research Centers (Part A); University Affiliated Facilities (UAFs; Part B); and Communi-

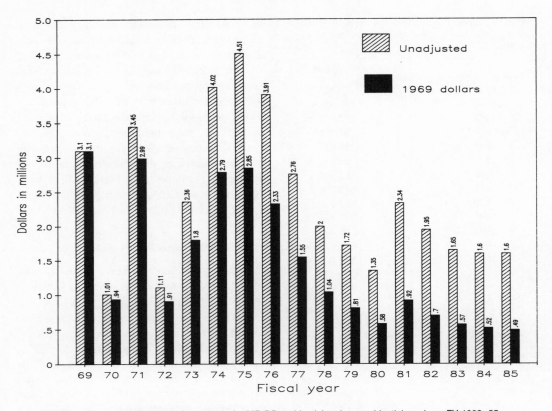

Figure 33.   Federal CHAMPUS payments for MR/DD residential and nonresidential services: FY 1969–85.

ty Facilities (Part C). Between FY 1965 and FY 1967, $27.005 million was federally obligated for the planning and erection of 12 mental retardation research centers. UAFs expended a total of $38.571 million in construction funds between FY 1965 and FY 1973, of which $1.622 million stemmed from state formula grant appropriations budgeted pursuant to PL 88-164's successor legislation, the Developmental Disabilities Services and Facilities Construction Act of 1970—PL 91-517. Community facility construction funds expended between FY 1965 and FY 1970 totaled $90.241 million. (Consult Chapter 7 for an extended discussion of PL 88-164, and for a presentation of annually budgeted expenditures for all construction and staffing grant activities).

PL 91-517 significantly expanded the scope and purposes of PL 88-164, emphasizing planning and the provision of state formula

grants for services. Although formula grant funds could be used under PL 91-517 for construction purposes, little money was actually spent in the states for this purpose. The substitution of the term "developmental disability," for "mental retardation," as in PL 88-164, also marked the addition of two new target populations, in addition to persons with mental retardation, eligible to receive services: persons with cerebral palsy and persons with epilepsy. One key component of the definition of developmental disability, in addition to the requirement that the disability manifest itself prior to age 18, was derived from Title II of the Social Security Act. In 1956, Title II had authorized trust fund benefits to be paid to eligible "Adult Disabled Children" beginning in 1956, and it defined disability in terms of an individual's inability to engage in "substantial gainful activity" over an extended and continuous period of time (12 months).

Table 16. CHAMPUS Program for persons with MR/DD: FY 1969–85 (dollars are in thousands)

FY	Number of residential days paid	Government cost (residential)	Number of claims (nonresidential)	Government cost (nonresidential)	Number of total claims	Total MR/DD payments
1969					8,406	$3,069
1970					2,691	$1,010
1971					8,368	$3,451
1972					2,451	$1,109
1973					4,817	$2,363
1974					8,382	$4,021
1975	—				9,941	$4,507
1976					8,686	$3,914
1977					5,705	$2,755
1978	20,550	$1,349	1,400	$650	3,688	$1,999
1979	21,736	$1,233	1,105	$486	3,149	$1,720
1980	16,421	$871	1,108	$481	2,614	$1,353
1981	15,012	$1,545	941	$793	2,145	$2,339
1982	20,878	$1,276	819	$671	1,667	$1,947
1983	24,926	$1,297	457	$312	1,409	$1,649
1984	25,612	$1,297	393	$312	1,350	$1,598
1985 (e)[a]	25,612	$1,297	393	$312	1,350	$1,598

Source: U.S. Department of Defense, CHAMPUS Office, Aurora, Colorado (R. Barnett, Chief, Statistics Branch, personal communication, August 23, 1983; and V. Nolan, personal communication, November 16, 1984).

[a]Estimated.

The Developmental Disabilities Assistance and Bill of Rights Act of 1975, PL 94-103, authorized a 3-year extension of state formula grants to assist in planning and implementing programs for children and adults with developmental disabilities; like PL 91-517, it also continued operational support for UAFs. A new special project authority was added to the legislation and for the first time persons with autism were eligible for services. Also notable was a provision that a DD state plan had to develop and incorporate a "deinstitutionalization and institutional reform" plan. The deinstitutionalization plan had to include a

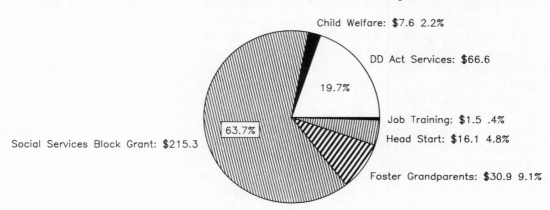

Child Welfare: $7.6 2.2%

DD Act Services: $66.6

19.7%

Job Training: $1.5 .4%

Head Start: $16.1 4.8%

Foster Grandparents: $30.9 9.1%

63.7%

Social Services Block Grant: $215.3

Total: $338 Million

Figure 34. Federal funding for MR/DD human development services: FY 1985. (Dollars are in millions.)

provision protecting employee interests. States were also required to develop evaluation systems, but this requirement was later dropped. It was also stipulated in the new law that the term "developmental disability" would be the subject of an independent contractual study to gauge its appropriateness.

In 1978, the act was revised by PL 95-602, the Rehabilitation, Comprehensive Services, and Developmental Disabilities Amendments. The new DD definition shifted its focus to functionality from category of disability, and it emphasized the severity and chronicity of the functional impairments. Changes in the program included the revised definition; a shift of emphasis from planning to provision of "priority services"; and increased authorization levels for state Protection and Advocacy systems. The act also specified that the state DD Council and the administering agency were to "jointly" develop a state DD plan. The composition of the state DD planning council was also modified to allow at least one-half, instead of one-third, of its members to be consumer representatives. The remainder was to be made up of provider and state agency representatives.

PL 97-35, the Omnibus Budget Reconciliation Act of 1981, extended the DD Act (PL 95-602) for 3 years. In 1984, Congress enacted legislation, PL 98-527, the Developmental Disabilities Act Amendments of 1984. In the 1984 legislation, the statement of overall purposes of the act, Section 101(b), was amended to include the purposes of: 1) assisting states to ensure that individuals with developmental disabilities receive the services necessary for them to achieve their maximum potential through increased independence, productivity, and integration into the community; and 2) to establish and operate a system to coordinate, plan, monitor, and evaluate services to persons with developmental disabilities. Definitions were added for "independence," "integration," "employment-related activities," and "supported employment" and the definitions of "services activities," "priority services," "satellite centers," and "university affiliated facility" are modified.

The federal share of all projects assisted under the state grant program was not to exceed 75% of the aggregate costs of all such projects (90% of the aggregate costs of projects in poverty areas). (Previously, these federal matching limits were set on *each* project assisted under the state grant program.)

Section 108 of PL 98-527 required the Secretary of Health and Human Services and the Secretary of Education to establish an interagency committee to coordinate and plan activities conducted by federal departments and agencies for persons with developmental disabilities; in Section 122, there were changes related to the state planning council's access to records, and a provision that no more than 25% of a state's grant funds may be allocated to the state agency for provision of services. Also, a new comprehensive statewide plan for provision of priority services must be developed by the second year of funding after enactment of this bill, and the state plan must provide assurances that the state will provide the state planning council with a copy of each report on the annual survey of an ICF/MR in the state.

In Section 123, the requirement for a habilitation plan for each developmentally disabled person assisted under the state plan was amended to include, in the statement of long-term habilitation goals, the increase or support of independence, productivity, and integration into the community. The requirement concerning the composition of the state planning councils, Section 124, was amended to specify that they shall include representatives of state agencies administering programs under the Rehabilitation Act of 1973, the Education of the Handicapped Act, Title XIX (Medicaid) of the Social Security Act, any UAF or satellite center in the state, and the state protection and advocacy system. This section also specified that the "groups concerned with services for the developmentally disabled" that must be represented on the council are "private nonprofit" groups.

Part C, Section 142, added several new requirements concerning state protection and advocacy systems. State systems must have authority to provide information on and referral to programs and services addressing the needs of persons with developmental disabilities. It was also required that the protection and advocacy system have access to the records of persons with developmental disabilities living in residential facilities if a complaint has been received on behalf of such person and if such person does not have a legal guardian or if the state is the legal guardian. The state must furnish to the protection and advocacy system a copy of the survey report on each ICF/MR within the state.

In Part D, UAFs, a new section (151) restated the corresponding provision in Section 101, and added to the purpose the dissemination of information that will increase and support the independence, productivity, and integration into the community of persons with developmental disabilities. Section 152 made several

amendments to the provisions concerning grants for UAFs. Grants may be made for studies of the feasibility of establishing a UAF or satellite center in an unserved area, including the need for such a facility, and authority is eliminated for grants to assess needs for trained personnel. Authority for grants for service-related training was amended to specify persons whose training may be assisted; satellite centers may carry out all activities that may be carried out by a UAF; and grants may not be made to a new UAF or satellite center after FY 1985 unless a feasibility study and needs assessment for such a facility has been conducted. (See Table 17 for a breakdown of funding for FY 1969–85 in the areas just discussed.)

Section 3 required the DHHS secretary, within 6 months after the bill's enactment, to

Table 17. Developmental Disabilities Act funding summary, excluding construction: FY 1969–85 (dollars are in thousands)

FY	UAF Training Grants	State Formula Grants	Special Projects	Protection & Advocacy	Staffing Grants
1969					$8,358
1970					$10,990
1971		$11,215			$8,272
1972	$4,250	$19,919			$3,920
1973	$4,433	$26,674	$7,494		$3,384
1974	$4,335	$27,585	$8,275		
1975	$4,250	$28,176	$21,199		
1976	$4,250	$31,558	$18,432		
1977	$5,200	$33,058	$19,617		
1978	$6,500	$41,608	$19,567	$3,000	
1979	$7,420	$30,058	$12,568	$3,000	
1980	$7,000	$43,680	$4,756	$7,500	
1981	$7,400	$42,180	$2,500	$7,500	
1982	$7,200	$41,453	$2,500	$7,680	
1983	$7,500	$43,180	$2,500	$7,320	
1984	$7,800	$43,750	$2,447	$8,400	
1985	$9,000	$50,250	$2,700	$13,700	

Source: State Grant Program fiscal data for FY 1971–72 are from Braddock (1973, p. 103). All other data predating FY 1973 are from Braddock (1973, p. 137). DD state grants were used for construction projects in FY 1971–74. According to House appropriations hearings data, construction funding for these years was $1.796 million in FY 1972 (Office of Mental Retardation Coordination [ORMC], 1973, p. 65); $1.584 million in FY 1973 (OHI, 1975, p. 68). These funds are omitted from this table (see Chapter 7).

All fiscal data for FY 1973 and FY 1974 are from the FY 1975 House hearings (OHI, 1974). Data for FY 1976 are from the Office for Handicapped Individuals (OHI, 1977). Data for FY 1977 and FY 1978 are from FY 1979 House hearings (U.S. House of Representatives [House], 1978, p. 1139). Data for FY 1979–85 were obtained from the Budget Office of the Administration on Developmental Disabilities (Shirley Redmond, personal communication, December 12, 1984).

transmit a report to Congress making recommendations for improving services under the Medicaid program, and specifically under home and community-based waivers under Section 1915(c) of the Social Security Act.

Expenditure Trends   State Formula Grants were initially allocated under PL 91-517 in FY 1971, although FY 1972 was the first full year of funding. As illustrated in Figure 35, unadjusted budgetary increases were deployed for services from 1971 to 1977. A sizable increase was budgeted in FY 1978, followed immediately by a large reduction in FY 1979, beneath the FY 1977 level. A significant increase was again obligated in FY 1980, followed by essentially flat expenditure performance for FY 1981–84. In FY 1985, the program received a $50.25 million appropriation, a $6.5 million increase, nearly 15% above the FY 1984 level of $43.75 million.

Although the State Formula Grant Program has received a fairly large annual increase in appropriations five times since FY 1972, the program has been cut or essentially held at the previous year's funding level seven times. The inconsistent budgetary growth exhibited between FY 1973 and FY 1984 averaged only 6% per annum in unadjusted terms. In real economic terms, the picture is extremely bleak. The program's funding actually regressed 30% between FY 1973 and FY 1984. Expenditures in FY 1978, in fact, represented the high-water mark for the program on an adjusted basis; the FY 1978 figure was 47% higher than the sum budgeted for FY 1985.

Federal funding for the operation of UAFs was authorized with the passage of PL 91-517, the Developmental Disabilities Services and Facilities Construction Act. Funding of $4.25 million was initially deployed, and it

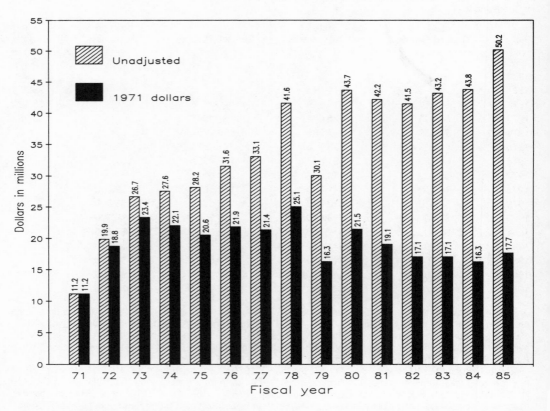

Figure 35.   Federal Developmental Disabilities Act funding for State Formula Grants, excluding construction: FY 1971–85.

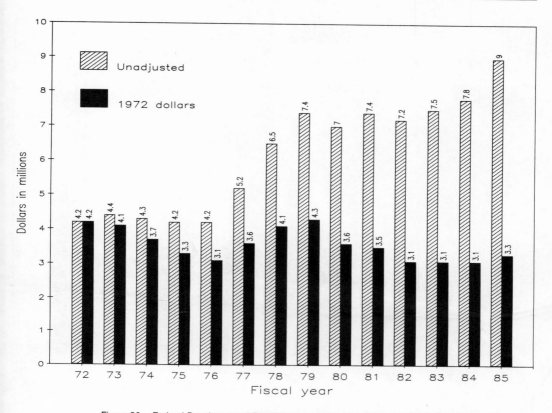

Figure 36.   Federal Developmental Disabilities Act funding for UAFs: FY 1972–85.

remained at that level through FY 1976. Between FY 1977 and FY 1979, funding increased on an unadjusted basis by an average of $1.1 million per annum to $7.4 million. It remained at about that level for the next 5 consecutive years through FY 1984. The FY 1985 appropriation was increased to $9 million. In FY 1984, 43 UAFs and satellites were receiving assistance and several new satellite UAFs were scheduled to begin operation in FY 1985.

In real economic terms, UAF funding fell annually between FY 1972 and FY 1976, increased slightly during FY 1977–79, and diminished from FY 1980 to FY 1984. The FY 1985 appropriation is an adjusted increase of 6.5%. UAF funding trends in unadjusted and real economic terms are presented in Figure 36.

The Protection and Advocacy program was authorized in the Comprehensive Rehabilita-

tion and Developmental Disabilities Services Act Amendments of 1978. The program received an initial appropriation of $3 million in FY 1978. Funding was increased to $7.5 million in FY 1980 and $7.68 million in FY 1982. Expenditures fell slightly in FY 1983 to $7.32 million, but an increase to $8.4 million was budgeted in FY 1984. Appropriations for FY 1985 jumped to $13.7 million, an unadjusted increase of 63% over the FY 1984 level (see Figure 37).

Funding for the Special Project authority has varied more widely on a year-to-year basis than any other DD Act–supported program. Initiated in FY 1973 at $7.49 million, funding for Special Projects almost tripled to $21.2 million in FY 1975. Funding ranged between $19.6 million and $12.6 million over the next 4 years, then plunged to $4.76 million in FY 1980, and $2.5 million in FY 1981. Spending was frozen at that level through FY 1984. A

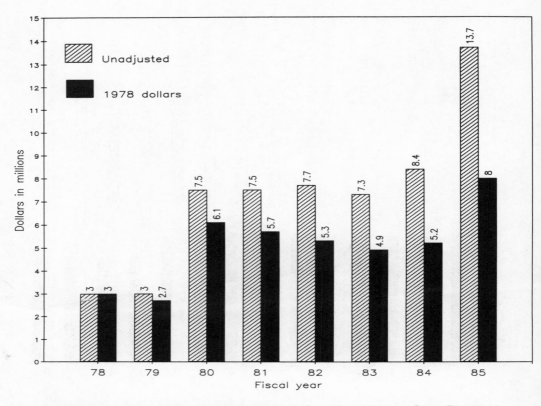

Figure 37.   Federal Developmental Disabilities Act funding for Protection and Advocacy Grants: FY 1978–85.

slight increase to $2.7 million was appropriated in FY 1985. In real economic terms, the budgeting of Special Project funds dropped every year between FY 1975 and FY 1984, as displayed in Figure 38. On an adjusted basis, the FY 1985 appropriation is an increase of 10% over the FY 1984 level.

Title XX, Social Services Block Grant
The term "social services" refers to a wide range of services to recipients or applicants for public assistance, to those previously receiving assistance, and to those likely to become applicants for or recipients of public assistance. The intent of Congress in extending services to potential welfare recipients was to prevent needy individuals from becoming dependent on welfare. Congress initially authorized the provision of social services to welfare recipients on a 50-50 reimbursement basis with the states. The Social Security Amendments of 1962 increased the federal matching ratio to

75%. In March of 1962, the DHEW Secretary announced a program policy change permitting federal financial participation to assist persons on conditional release from mental institutions. In 1972, due to growing concern over the rapidly escalating social services costs, a rider was attached to the State and Local Fiscal Assistance Act (PL 92-512), which placed a $2.5 billion ceiling on federal funding for social services. The rider required the states to spend at least 90% of their outlays on applicants for or recipients of federally assisted welfare payments. However, services to persons with mental retardation was one of the areas exempted from the 90% requirement.

The Social Services Amendments of 1974 (PL 93-647) consolidated Social Services Grants to the states under a new Title XX of the Social Security Act. Amendments in 1976 (PL 94-401) temporarily increased authorizations by $200 million annually to support

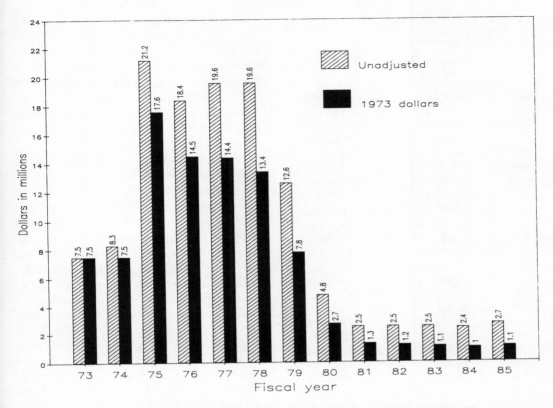

Figure 38.   Federal Developmental Disabilities Act funding for Special Projects: FY 1973–85.

child day care services, and eliminated the required state matching funds for outlays from this special allotment. In 1980, the Title XX program was significantly revised under PL 96-272. Among the major changes were: 1) permanent funding authorization increases over a 6-year period culminating in a FY 1985 ceiling of $3.3 billion; 2) restrictions on the amount of funds available for Title XX training activities; 3) a multiyear planning authority; and 4) a separate funding authority for Puerto Rico and territories. In FY 1982, Title XX was converted into the Social Services Block Grant under provisions of the Omnibus Budget Reconciliation Act of 1981 (PL 97-35). A state match was no longer required. (See Table 18 for a review of the funding for FY 1963–85.)

The Social Services Program has been an important source of funds for the development of community-based MR/DD services for 2

decades. However, except for a federally administered survey of MR/DD expenditures in FY 1973, and the data reported for FY 1977–84 in the study by Braddock et al. (1984), only rough agency estimates of MR/DD social services expenditures have been available.

Braddock (1973, p. 112) estimated social services expenditures to adult and Aid to Families with Dependent Children (AFDC) public assistance recipients between FY 1963 and FY 1972 as based on the prevalence of mental retardation among these recipients as determined by the National Center for Social Statistics. Mental retardation funding grew on an unadjusted basis from an estimated $1.85 million in FY 1963, to $113.9 million in FY 1973. During this period, total federal spending for social services advanced from $30 million to $1.885 billion. As just stated, such rapid funding growth in the "uncapped" program led Congress to legislate the $2.5 billion

Table 18. Estimated MR/DD funding under Title XX and the Social Services Block Grant: FY 1963–85 (dollars are in thousands)

FY	Total program funding	Estimated MR/DD reimbursements
1963	$30,341	$1,853
1964	$73,249	$4,780
1965	$113,845	$7,209
1966	$154,555	$9,815
1967	$235,528	$14,948
1968	$287,717	$18,358
1969	$286,726	$24,580
1970	$671,835	$43,017
1971	$750,007	$47,900
1972	$1,606,736	$102,900
1973	$1,885,566	$113,900
1974	$2,500,000	$123,119
1975	$2,500,000	$132,335
1976	$2,226,428	$141,552
1977	$2,335,332	$151,345
1978	$2,401,300	$178,125
1979	$2,853,529	$192,070
1980	$2,681,890	$241,725
1981	$2,991,000	$250,253
1982	$2,400,000	$202,889
1983	$2,675,000	$216,429
1984	$2,700,000	$212,041
1985	$2,725,000	$215,275

Source: Data for FY 1963–1973 are from Braddock (1973, p. 112). Data for FY 1977–1984 are based on the state-by-state expenditure analysis in Braddock, Hemp, and Howes (1984). FY 1974–76 data are estimated by interpolating between the estimated expenditure for FY 1973 and the actual FY 1977 figure from the Braddock et al. (1984) state-by-state study. MR/DD expenditures for FY 1985 were estimated by figuring the percentage of total Title XX funds that MR/DD expenditures constituted in the previous 5 years (average 7.9%) and then applying that percentage to the FY 1985 Social Services Block Grant appropriation.

ceiling on the Social Services Program, contained in the FY 1972 State and Local Fiscal Assistance Act, PL 92-512.

As illustrated in Figure 39, estimated spending for MR/DD services grew every year during FY 1973–81, although at a much slower rate than during FY 1963–72. Funding dropped in FY 1982, by 20%, but increased slightly in FY 1983–85.

In real economic terms, mental retardation funding grew every year from FY 1963 to FY

1973 and then plateaued over the next 6 years. The rate of regression in funding for MR/DD services (which began again in FY 1981 after the program's adjusted expenditure peak in FY 1980) was 36% from FY 1980 to FY 1985, or an average of 8% annually. This diminution represents significant regression in funding for MR/DD services in a key federal program.

Social Security Act as Amended: Child Welfare Services Since the passage of the original Social Security Act in 1935, the federal government has provided matching formula grants to state and local departments of public welfare for child welfare services. These services, authorized under Title IV, Part B, include casework and referral, foster family placement, arrangements for homemaker services, day care, and institutional care. In contrast to the AFDC and, for a time, the adult Social Services Program (Title XX), the Child Welfare Program appropriation has been closed-ended since FY 1968. Federal participation in the program has been less than 10% of combined federal-state-local expenditures. (See Table 19 for funding obligations for FY 1955–85.)

The Adoption Assistance and Child Welfare Act of 1980, PL 96-272, revised the allotment basis and tripled the program's budget. A principle objective of the revision was to expand adoption opportunities in lieu of foster care. Title IV, Part E of the act authorizes federal support for adoption subsidies.

Economic Opportunity Act of 1964 as Amended: Head Start Project Head Start was initially authorized under the Economic Opportunity Act of 1964, during the "War on Poverty." The program offers health, educational, nutritional, social, and other services to economically deprived preschool children. Project grants are made to local public agencies and nonprofit organizations to operate Head Start classes and services throughout the United States.

The Economic Opportunity Act Amendments of 1972, PL 92-424, directed the Secretary of HEW to establish policies and procedures designed to assure that "not less than

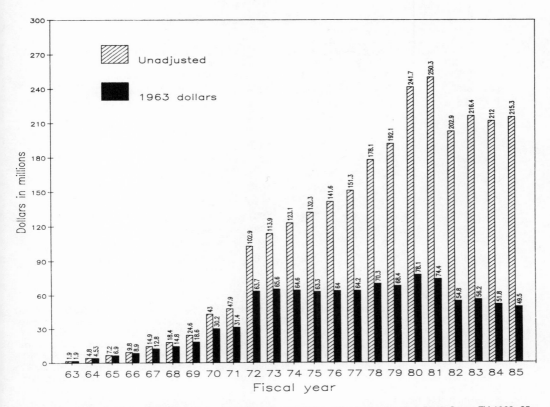

Figure 39. Estimated federal MR/DD reimbursements under Title XX and the Social Services Block Grant: FY 1963–85.

10 percent of the total number of enrollment opportunities in the nation in the Head Start Program shall be available for handicapped children." "Handicapped" was defined in the act according to provisions of the Education of the Handicapped Act, Section 602. The Community Services Act of 1974, PL 93-644, revised the requirement concerning handicapped child enrollments by stipulating that each state had to assure that 10% of enrollees were children with handicaps. (See Table 20 for estimated Head Start expenditures for FY 1965–85.)

Domestic Volunteer Service Act of 1973
The Foster Grandparent Program was first developed in FY 1966 by the Administration on Aging of HEW, and was funded by the Office of Economic Opportunity (OEO) in the executive office of the president. Its specific purpose has been two-fold—demonstrating the benefits of employing older persons and of enriching the social environments of institutionalized children and youth. The 1969 amendments to the Older Americans Act established the program by an act of Congress with both funding and administration carried out under HEW auspices.

The program has reached not only individuals with MR/DD, but also institutionalized mentally ill persons, dependent and neglected persons, physically handicapped individuals, and juvenile offenders. Administrative authority and operational support for the program were transferred from HEW to Action Agency in FY 1972. In 1973, Congress consolidated a variety of existing federal voluntary service programs with the enactment of the Domestic Volunteer Service Act (PL 93-113). This legislation created the Action Agency and authorized the Senior Companion Program, which was aimed at working with frail elderly persons.

Table 19. Child Welfare Program estimated mental retardation obligations: FY 1955–85 (dollars are in thousands)

FY	Total obligations	Estimated MR $	FY	Total obligations	Estimated MR $
1955	$6,900	$483	1971	$46,000	$3,220
1956	$6,900	$483	1972	$46,000	$3,220
1957	$7,900	$553	1973	$46,000	$1,748
1958	$9,500	$665	1974	$47,500	$1,805
1959	$11,900	$833	1975	$50,000	$1,900
1960	$13,000	$910	1976	$52,500	$1,995
1961	$13,700	$959	1977	$56,500	$2,147
1962	$17,800	$1,246	1978	$56,500	$2,147
1963	$26,100	$1,827	1979	$56,500	$2,147
1964	$28,800	$2,016	1980	$56,150	$2,133
1965	$34,200	$2,394	1981	$163,550	$6,214
1966	$39,700	$2,779	1982	$156,326	$5,940
1967	$45,700	$3,199	1983	$156,326	$5,940
1968	$46,871	$3,281	1984	$165,000	$6,270
1969	$46,855	$3,280	1985	$200,000	$7,600
1970	$46,000	$3,220			

Source: Data for FY 1955–73 are from Braddock (1973, p. 115). Mental retardation estimates are based on a 1963 study by the U.S. Children's Bureau (1963) reporting that 7% of child welfare recipients nationwide were mentally retarded. In 1981, the bureau published another study (U.S. Children's Bureau, 1981) based on FY 1977 data and indicated that 3.8% of Child Welfare Program recipients were mentally retarded. To determine estimated mental retardation expenditures, the 7% figure was applied to total child welfare obligations from FY 1955 to FY 1973; from FY 1974 to FY 1985, the 3.8% estimate was used. Total program expenditures for FY 1974–85 were provided by the Budget Director of the U.S. Children's Bureau (J. Rich, personal communication, November 16, 1984).

House subcommittee hearings on "Supplemental Appropriation to Combat Mental Retardation" (House, 1963, p. 45) reported that "an estimated ten percent" of the 423,000 children receiving child welfare services in FY 1962 were mentally retarded. There is little doubt that significant numbers of children with mental retardation and their families benefit from this program; but accurately determining the numbers served, the budgeted expenditures, and the variable costs is not possible at this time.

Amendments to the act in 1976 authorized the Action Agency to allow individuals with MR/DD to participate in the Foster Grandparent Program after they reached the age of 21. In 1978, with the passage of the Comprehensive Older Americans Act (PL 95-478), the Foster Grandparent Program was extended for an additional 3 years and its authorization was consolidated with the Senior Companion Program. The legislation also raised a stipend that participants could receive from $1.60/hour to $2.00/hour.

The Older Americans Act Amendments of 1979 (PL 96-143) established the "Helping Hand" Program, designed to increase the ability of elderly and handicapped persons to remain in the community and prevent isolation and institutionalization. The Helping Hand Program was to be coordinated with the state's developmental disability protection and advocacy system.

Between 71% and 64% of all children served under the Foster Grandparents Program during FY 1966–73 period were mentally retarded or developmentally disabled residents of state institutions. Since FY 1974, that percentage has dropped to an estimated 55%. In FY 1971, 6,240 children with MR/DD were provided services. In FY 1984, the estimated number of children with MR/DD served was 35,468. There were 18,425 grandparents involved in the program in FY 1984, up from 4,400 in FY 1971.

Funding for the Foster Grandparent Program increased during FY 1966–71, from $5.1 million to $10.4 million. In FY 1972, funding more than doubled to $25 million. In FY 1975–76, funds budgeted increased to

Table 20. Estimated expenditures for children with mental retardation in Project Head Start: FY 1965–85 (dollars are in thousands)

FY	Head Start Total budget	% MR services	Cost factor	Estimated MR $
1965	$96,400			
1966	$198,900			
1967	$349,200			
1968	$316,200			
1969	$333,900			
1970	$325,700			
1971	$360,000			
1972	$376,317			
1973	$400,700			
1974	$403,900	0.75	x2	$6,059
1975	$403,900	0.75	x2	$6,059
1976	$441,000	0.75	x2	$6,615
1977	$625,000	0.75	x2	$9,375
1978	$625,000	0.75	x2	$9,375
1979	$625,000	0.75	x2	$9,375
1980	$735,000	0.75	x2	$11,025
1981	$818,000	0.75	x2	$12,270
1982	$911,700	0.75	x2	$13,676
1983	$912,000	0.75	x2	$13,680
1984	$995,750	0.75	x2	$14,936
1985	$1,075,059	0.75	x2	$16,126

Source: Data for FY 1965–72 are from Braddock (1973, p. 69). Total budget data for FY 1973–85 are from Administrative Records, Head Start Budget Bureau (D. Klafein, personal communication, December 11, 1984). Service utilization data on the full-year handicapped child program indicated that 6.3% of all handicapped children served in 1981 were mentally retarded. Handicapped children made up 11.99% of all Head Start children served in FY 1980 (Head Start Bureau, 1982). Although the percentage of children varies from year to year, .75% was used as a reasonable estimate (.063 × .1199).

An earlier study in 1970 reported that 1.3% of Head Start children served had a "learning problem or MR," and an additional .2% had "cerebral dysfunction or CP." In this table, estimated mental retardation expenditures are presented for FY 1974–1985. A few children with mental retardation were served prior to the 10% legislative mandate for handicapped child enrollment in FY 1973, but their numbers were very small. Even in 1980, only 2,753 out of 364,400 children were identified in Project Head Start nationally as having mental retardation as their "primary or most disabling condition" (Head Start Bureau, 1982, p. 12, note 2).

The estimated mental retardation expenditure figures were, however, predicated on the assumption that providing services to a substantially disabled child with mental retardation in Project Head Start is twice as expensive as providing similar services to non–mentally retarded children (Kakalik et al., 1981).

$28.3 million and for FY 1977–79, the figure was $34.9 million. Appropriations for the program were raised to $46.9 million in FY 1980, and gradually raised to $49.7 million in FY 1984. The appropriation for FY 1985 was $56.1 million, an increase of 13% over the FY 1984 level. (Estimated funding for MR/DD services for FY 1966–85 is presented in Table 21.)

In real economic terms, the funding for children with MR/DD declined slightly during FY 1968–70, more than doubled in FY 1972, and then leveled off. The program has benefited from sporadic large annual increases in funding, but the overall trend from FY 1973 to FY 1985 was generally regressive, as depicted in Figure 40.

Department of Labor Services   The Comprehensive Employment and Training Act (CETA) supported job training activities for persons with MR/DD from FY 1967 to FY 1982. Handicapped persons were eligible to participate in most CETA programs under services targeted specifically to handicapped individuals and under certain programs provided for the "economically disadvantaged" and "unemployed."

Although many individuals with handicaps were eligible to participate in CETA programs by virtue of inadequate income and lack of employability, specific recognition of the employment and training needs of persons with handicaps was not included in the statute until the CETA amendments of 1978 (PL 95-524). This legislation required state and local prime sponsors to include in their master and annual plans, descriptions of employment services provided to individuals with handicaps. Representatives of handicapped persons' interests were also required to be included on the state employment and training councils, and all

CETA state and local prime sponsors and subcontractors were required to prohibit discrimination on the basis of handicap.

In addition, under Title III of the act, a new section, 306, was added which called for the establishment of programs to train personnel working with and assisting handicapped individuals. Also, Congress adopted the Job Training Partnership Act of 1982, which went into effect on October 1, 1983.

(See Table 22 for funding levels of four U.S. Department of Labor [DOL] MR/DD job training projects. The figures presented in the table do not include any estimates of DOL-funded "CETA-type" state and locally organized training efforts involving MR/DD persons. The extent to which persons with

Table 21. Foster Grandparent Program estimated expenditures: FY 1966–85 (dollars are in thousands)

FY	Total obligations	MR/DD funds	Total grandparents	Total children served
1966	$5,108	$3,576	782	1,955
1967	$5,840	$3,854	2,000	5,000
1968	$9,575	$6,224	4,000	10,000
1969	$8,973	$5,832	4,100	10,250
1970	$8,817	$6,172	4,200	10,500
1971	$10,403	$7,386	4,400	11,000
1972	$25,000	$17,974	10,036	25,090
1973	$25,000	$16,000	9,873	24,683
1974	$25,000	$16,000	12,193	30,483
1975	$28,287	$15,557	13,600	34,000
1976	$28,347	$15,590	13,900	34,750
1977	$34,000	$18,700	16,000	40,000
1978	$34,900	$19,195	16,250	40,625
1979	$34,900	$19,195	16,640	41,600
1980	$46,900	$25,795	16,929	42,323
1981	$48,400	$26,620	18,093	63,326
1982	$46,079	$26,620	18,093	63,326
1983	$48,400	$26,620	18,350	64,225
1984	$49,700	$27,720	18,425	64,488
1985	$56,100	$30,855		

Source: Data for FY 1966–1973 are from Braddock (1973, p. 135), and are based on the actual percentage of children with MR/DD served among all children served in the Foster Grandparent Program during these years. Data for FY 1975–85 were provided by the Chief of the Foster Grandparent Program Branch, Office of Older American Volunteer Programs, Action Agency (J. Kenyon, personal communications, July 14, 1983, and November 29, 1984). Kenyon estimated that 55% of the Foster Grandparent Program's activities annually over the past 10 years have consistently involved serving individuals with MR/DD. Estimated MR/DD funds are 55% of total program obligations for this period. The program was unable to provide more precise client data.

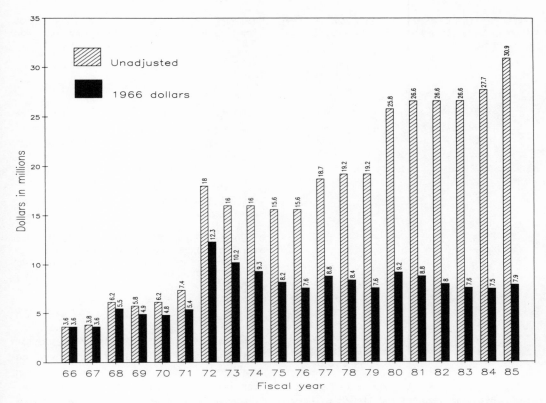

Figure 40.   Estimated funding for services to persons with mental retardation or developmental disabilities under the Foster Grandparent Program: FY 1966–85.

SUPPLEMENTARY FEDERAL PROGRAM INFORMATION

Funding for the three programs presented in this section is presented for informational purposes only. This funding has not been included in the computations that form the basis of the analysis of federal government MR/DD expenditures in Chapter 9.

Social Security Act, Title V, Section 508: Maternity and Infant Care   Enacted on October 24, 1963, the Maternal and Child Health and Mental Retardation Planning Act of 1963 (PL 88-156) was the first piece of federal legislation implementing a major recommendation of the President's Panel on Mental Retardation (1962). Part 4 of the act authorized special project grants for maternity and infant

care projects "to help reduce the incidence of mental retardation caused by complications associated with child-bearing." These grants, incorporated as Section 508 of the Social Security Act, were extended by the 1967 Social Security Act Amendments (PL 90-248).

In 1972, a 1-year extender, PL 92-445, continued the Maternity and Infant Care Program through June 30, 1973 (see Table A for funding for FY 1964–73). The thrust of this program was to reduce infant and maternal mortality and morbidity by providing, through state health agencies, matching federal funds to help provide necessary health care to high risk mothers and infants. Many handicapping conditions associated with a prenatal or neonatal causality, such as mental retardation, are preventable with appropriate care like that provided under the auspices of maternity and infant care projects. In FY 1970, 117,000 maternity patients were served and 42,000 in-

Table 22. U.S. Department of Labor Job Training Program for MR/DD persons: FY 1967–1985 (dollars are in thousands)

FY	Funding for four MR/DD DOL projects
1967	$593
1968	$0
1969	$0
1970	$252
1971	$222
1972	$395
1973	$749
1974	$700
1975	$769
1976	$1,123
1977	$1,208
1978	$1,299
1979	$1,346
1980	$1,387
1981	$1,471
1982	$1,280
1983	$1,472
1984	$1,472
1985	$1,472

Source: At the author's request, the DOL identified four relevant MR/DD job training projects. The figures presented are the yearly aggregates for the projects' funding. Funding levels for the "On the Job Training" Project of the National Association for Retarded Citizens (NARC) were obtained from the Office of Strategic Planning and Policy Development, Office of Special National Level Programs, Employment and Training Administration (B. Rann, Handicapped Coordinator, personal communication, July 21, 1983). About 90% of all funding presented in this table are for the NARC project, which has been operating continuously since 1967 (3 years' funding was received in 1967).

Goodwill Industries of America's national office has operated a special training project for MR/DD persons continuously since FY 1976 at a constant estimated sum of $276,000/year. Estimates were provided by Goodwill's Director of "Projects with Industry" (J. Scott, personal communication, July 21, 1983).

The Electronic Industries Foundation, according to its Project Director (C. Dunlap, personal communication, July 21, 1983), has supported DD training continuously since FY 1978 at an annual level of about $35,000.

A fourth project identified by the DOL involves staff training in rehabilitation facilities, including training of staff in state MR/DD residential institutions. This project is operated by the National Association of Rehabilitation Facilities. All figures were updated for FY 1985 appropriations by Rann (personal communication, November 21, 1984).

Table A. Social Security Act, Title V, Section 508, special project grants for maternity and infant care (MIC): FY 1964–73 (dollars are in thousands)

FY	MIC obligations
1964	$4,683
1965	$9,528
1966	$24,156
1967	$27,744
1968	$29,645
1969	$36,000
1970	$36,600
1971	$38,565
1972	$43,428
1973(e)[a]	$47,232

Source: The source of these data is Braddock (1973, p. 87), based on records of the Finance Division, Maternal and Child Health Service, Department of Health, Education, and Welfare.
[a]Estimated.

fants received care. Although the program was phased out in FY 1974, states were encouraged to incorporate maternity and infant care projects into their state health plans (Secretary's Committee on Mental Retardation, 1971, pp. 18–19).

Title XIX: Early and Periodic Screening, Diagnosis, and Treatment   Early and Periodic Screening, Diagnosis, and Treatment (EPSDT) was authorized by the Social Security Act Amendments of 1967, PL 90-248, Section 1905 (a)(4)(D). The act amended Title XIX of the Social Security Act to provide for early and periodic screening, diagnosis, and treatment of very young children of the poor. A requirement in the Social Security Act Amendments of 1972 to require a penalty reduction in the AFDC funds a state could receive if EPSDT was not "properly" implemented was repealed by the Omnibus Budget Reconciliation Act of 1981.

There are very little data available on the program and none are readily available specific to persons with MR/DD. In Table B, "children with referable conditions" include those with diagnosed problems in vision, hearing, speech, and in general physical and mental development.

Table B. Title XIX-Medicaid, EPSDT Services: FY 1975–79 (dollars are in thousands)

FY	No. of children screened	No. of children screened with referable conditions	Screening reimbursements
1975	1,800,000	900,000	$33,700
1976	2,000,000	1,000,000	$46,800
1977	2,100,000	1,100,000	$51,900
1978	2,000,000	1,000,000	$47,600
1979	2,000,000	1,000,000	$48,200

Source: Bureau of Data Management and Strategy, Health Care Financing Administration (D. Muse, director, personal communication, August 11, 1983). Data for FY 1980–84 were not available.

PL 93-151: Immunization Grants The Center for Disease Control administers a project grant program designed to help states reduce the communicability of disease. This program had a major impact on the prevention of diseases that can lead to mental retardation and other developmental disabilities, such as rubella, measles, and poliomyelitis. State grant funds expended under the auspices of the program are presented in Table C.

Table C. State grants for immunization projects: FY 1977–84 (dollars are in thousands)

FY	Funds obligated
1977	$18,494
1978	$32,970
1979	$46,883
1980	$30,363
1981	$30,713
1982	$34,715
1983	$39,260
1984	$41,889

Source: Administrative records, Center for Disease Control, Atlanta, Georgia.

Chapter 4

Personnel Training Programs

THE FEDERAL GOVERNMENT has been involved in the training of specialists in mental retardation and developmental disabilities for more than 30 years. The mission is divisible into four general categories of activity: 1) training of special educators, 2) training of rehabilitative personnel, 3) training of human development services personnel in University Affiliated Facility (UAF) Programs, and 4) training of biomedical and health services personnel. The fourth category includes training sponsored by the National Institutes of Health (NIH) and the Maternal and Child Health Services in the Department of Health and Human Services (DHHS). Special education and vocational rehabilitation training is administered by the Office of Special Education and Rehabilitative Services in the U.S. Department of Education. Figure 41 illustrates the FY 1985 funding configuration for MR/DD training sponsored by the federal government.

Federal support for the training of personnel in mental retardation began in FY 1954, with the initial expenditure of funds for the training of neurological specialists at the National Institute of Neurological Diseases and Blindness (NINDB). Congressman Fogarty's subcommittee identified the training of personnel as a major need in budget hearings during 1955. Soon thereafter, training budgets at NINDB and the Office of Education grew rapidly. In 1956, the Office of Vocational Rehabilitation began supporting workshops and seminars on the rehabilitation of mentally retarded persons. In 1958, Congress enacted PL 85-926.

This legislation, introduced by Congressman George McGovern, authorized a training program for teachers of children with mental retardation. It is the forerunner of the modern Special Education Personnel Preparation Program in the U.S. Department of Education.

After the 1962 issuance of the recommendations of the President's Panel on Mental Retardation, training activities expanded substantially in scope and depth. President Kennedy signed legislation creating the National Institute of Child Health and Human Development (NICHD) in 1962. In 1963, PL 88-164 extended and expanded the teacher training component established under PL 85-926. The National Institute of Mental Health (NIMH) also implemented the Hospital In-Service Training Program (HIST). The HIST Program operated for 13 years, FY 1964–77. In FY 1973, it reached 111 state MR/DD institutions.

The health services training mission was strengthened in FY 1967, with the budgeting of Section 511 training funds designed to improve the competencies of various health services personnel working with mothers and children. University Affiliated Facilities have been the principal recipients of these monies, receiving $13–$18 million every year since FY 1972. UAFs have also been the recipients of federal funds, since 1971, associated with personnel training activities under the Developmental Disabilities Act. During FY 1972–85, between $4.25 and $9 million was expended annually for general UAF administrative operations. (See Chapter 3 for a dis-

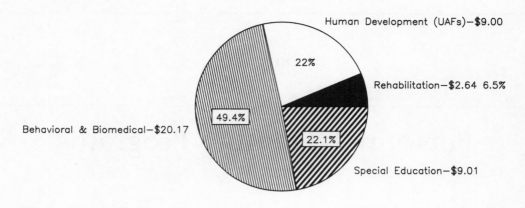

Total: $40.82 Million

Figure 41.   Federal spending for MR/DD training programs: FY 1985. (Dollars are in millions.)

cussion of the Developmental Disabilities Act's UAF Program administered under Part B of PL 88-164 as Amended.)

The general unadjusted trend in federal MR/DD training funding moved strongly upward between FY 1960 and FY 1972, as Figure 42 illustrates. Overall training support was flat from FY 1973 to FY 1980. During FY 1981–83, however, support fell 17%, due to substantial cutbacks in training of rehabilitation personnel and in Section 511 funding. Appropriation levels for FY 1985 rebounded training funds to a projected level 11% above the FY 1983 figure. In real economic terms, training funds advanced consistently upward every year from FY 1963 to FY 1972, except for FY 1970–71. Thereafter, training expenditures fell equally rapidly. Total training funding for FY 1985 was only 25% of the peak real funding level in FY 1972; and, along with the FY 1984 figure, it represented the smallest spending commitment for training in 22 years.

The rest of the chapter describes federal expenditures for each individual program under the aforementioned broad training categories. Each program's discussion contains: 1) an overview of the program, 2) a table displaying the MR/DD expenditures and other available program data, 3) the source of the data, and 4) for the major programs, a discussion of the expenditure trends over the history of the program.

TRAINING OF SPECIAL EDUCATION PERSONNEL

PL 88-164 as Amended (Title VI, Part D)

PL 85-926 authorized an initial appropriation of $1 million in FY 1960 for the preparation of professional personnel in the education of persons with mental retardation. On October 31, 1963, the Mental Retardation Facilities and Community Mental Health Centers Construction Act (PL 80-164) was signed into law. Title III, Section 301 of this act amended PL 85-926 and expanded the program to include not only mental retardation teacher training, but also training of teachers of emotionally disturbed, speech impaired, and physically handicapped children and youth. Title III also authorized support for research and for training of future college teachers.

Subsequent amendments to the act, including PL 91-230, Title VI D, in 1970, expanded the training program. The 1967 amendments (PL 90-170) added provisions for training physical education and recreation personnel.

Table 23 shows the funding patterns for the training of special education personnel for FY 1960–85. Data collection over the past 24

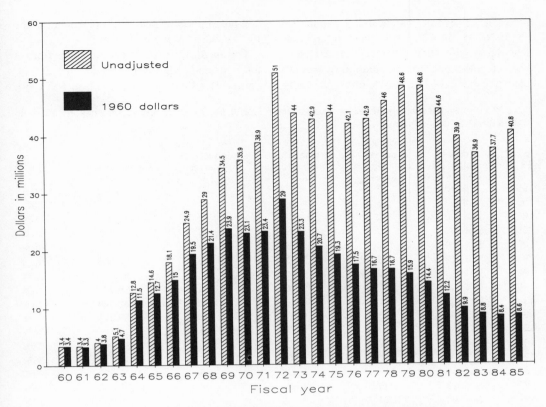

Figure 42.   Federal expenditures for MR/DD training programs: FY 1960–85.

years has followed three principle formats. From FY 1960 to FY 1971, data on mental retardation training was collected categorically in the Division of Personnel Preparation within the Bureau of Education for the Handicapped. All mental retardation data in Table 23 therefore are clearly identifiable from inspection of project grant proposals submitted by institutions of higher education and state education agencies. In FY 1971, $4 million was granted to 16 universities as "program support grants," rather than the traditional categorical traineeship grants.

In FY 1972, the Special Education Training Division moved entirely to program assistance grants as the funding mechanism. This made it technically impossible to precisely delineate trainees according to distinct areas of handicapping condition. Over the next several years, however, there are no data to support the notion that substantially fewer training programs had a mental retardation focus. In data submitted to Congress as a part of the FY 1974 and also FY 1977 congressional hearings on the HEW budget, it was stated that funding levels for mental retardation training programs remained at continuing high levels, even though a noncategorical funding mechanism had been adopted.

> . . . it is our best judgment from review of proposals received that the number of teachers being trained for mental retardation has not diminished. . . . and funds allocated have not been reduced. (Office for Handicapped Individuals [OHI], 1976, p. 24)

In FY 1977, funding and data collection emphases shifted to "severely handicapped" and "mildly and moderately handicapped" personnel training. The mental retardation expenditure estimates in Table 23 refer only to funds

Analytical Profiles

allocated for severely handicapped training in
FY 1976–85. In FY 1983, the funding and
data reporting strategy changed once again.
The categories now are preparation of special
education personnel at the B.A./M.A. level;

and preparation of leadership personnel at the
Ph.D. and post-doctoral level.

On an unadjusted basis, the budgeting of
total special education training funds advanced steadily from $1 million in FY 1960,

Table 23.   Training of special education personnel under Title VI, Part D, PL 85-926 as Amended: FY 1960–85
(dollars are in thousands)

FY	Total program $	No. of higher education institutions	Estimated no. of traineeships	No. of state education agencies	Estimated MR $	% MR $
1960	$985	16	177	23	$985	100%
1961	$993	18	164	41	$993	100%
1962	$2,492	20	160	46	$997	40%
1963	$12,993	19	163	48	$996	40%
1964	$14,499	108	2,357	50	$6,419	49%
1965	$19,500	153	2,506	50	$6,569	45%
1966	$24,500	162	3,110	52	$7,658	39%
1967	$24,500	177	3,816	53	$8,891	36%
1968	$29,700	177	4,521	53	$8,494	35%
1969	$29,700	193	6,366	53	$9,382	32%
1970	$32,491	200	6,171	55	$10,391	35%
1971	$34,645	207	4,909	55	$10,500	32%
1972	$37,700	210	5,100	56	$10,500	30%
1973	$37,655	215	4,830	56	$10,920	29%
1974	$39,615	225	4,529	56	$10,240	26%
1975	$37,700	225	3,146	55	$10,240	27%
1976	$40,375	225	2,691	55	$9,440	23%
1977	$45,375	225	3,143	55	$8,075	18%
1978	$45,375		2,991		$9,431	21%
1979	$55,375		2,658		$8,975	16%
1980	$55,375		2,998		$7,975	14%
1981	$43,500		3,461		$8,996	21%
1982	$49,300		3,461		$10,385	21%
1983	$49,300		3,461		$7,284	15%
1984	$55,540		2,735		$8,205	15%
1985	$61,000		2,735		$9,010	15%

Source: Total program expenditures for FY 1960–1973 are from Braddock (1973, p. 52); data for FY 1974–
1985 are from the Budget Office, Office of Special Education (OSE), U.S. Department of Education (B. Wolfe,
personal communication, November, 1984). FY 1985 figures are actual appropriations. The number of higher
education institutions and state education agencies for FY 1960–77 are from the FY 1979 House appropriations
hearings on the HEW budget (U.S. House of Representatives [House], 1978). Estimated mental retardation
fiscal data for FY 1960–73 are from FY 1976 House hearings on the HEW budget (Office for Handicapped
Individuals [OHI], 1975, p. 65).

Mental retardation data for FY 1976–85 are obligations for training for personnel working with "severely
handicapped" persons. The major focus of this training is for severe to profound MR/DD (OSE, J. Siantz,
personal communication, November 13, 1983). Traineeship data are from the FY 1979 House hearings for FY
1960–73 (House, 1978). Traineeship data for 1974–75 are projected from the FY 1973 figures. Traineeship
data for FY 1976–85 are from OSE, Department of Education (J. Siantz, personal communication, November
13, 1983), and refer to traineeships under the Severely Handicapped Training Program ($3,000 per trainee).

In FY 1983, institutions of higher education were given the authority to set the traineeship stipend levels. In
prior years, the stipends were fixed by the OSE. The FY 1984 budget figure is a *pro rata* projection of the FY
1983 actual figures for severely handicapped training, based on the actual total appropriations for Title VI D for
FY 1984.

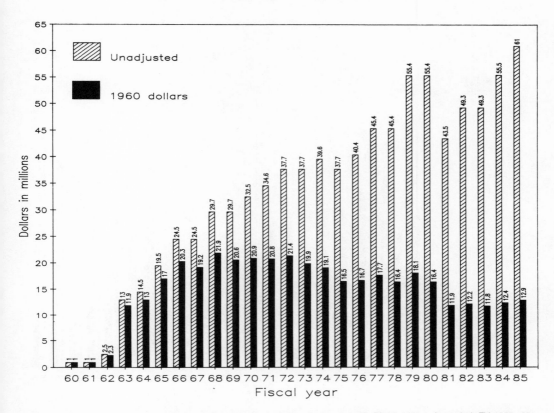

Figure 43.   Federal funding for the training of special education personnel under PL 85-926 as Amended: FY 1960–85.

to \$37.7 million in FY 1972. Thereafter, funding on an adjusted basis fell slightly, although the dominant trend since FY 1976 is that of a plateau. Total Part D funding for all special education training activity was \$6.1 million less in FY 1983 than in FY 1979. However, in the last 2 years, there has been a significant recovery of funds and the FY 1985 appropriation is 24% over the FY 1983 level, as illustrated in Figure 43.

In real economic terms, mental retardation training funding is in retrenchment. Between FY 1964 and FY 1967, program funding advanced and sustained the advance through FY 1970. Thereafter, 7 consecutive years of diminution followed, cutting real funding in half by FY 1977. After a 1-year increase in FY 1978, the decline continued through FY 1983, again reducing the level of real expenditure approximately in half. The Office of Special

Education estimated a slight increase in FY 1985, as illustrated in Figure 44.

PL 90-35: Education Professions Development Act (terminated)

Discretionary project grant funds were deployed under the Education Professions Development Act (EPDA) between FY 1969 and FY 1973. Funds were used for training and retraining regular classroom teachers to work with handicapped children. Total annual funding for the entire program ranged from \$113.6 million in FY 1969 to \$125.2 million in FY 1973. Between 3% and 6% of these funds were expended in projects concerned with the education of handicapped children. Braddock (1973, p. 65) indicated that EPDA staff estimated that half of the funds obligated for special projects for handicapped children and youth were in support of MR/DD activities.

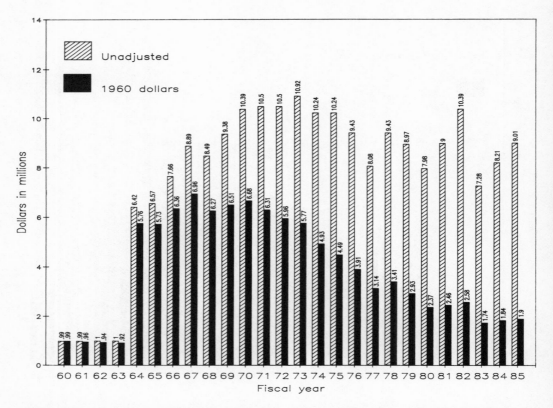

Figure 44. Estimated mental retardation expenditures for the training of special education personnel under PL 88-164, Title VI D: FY 1960–85.

TRAINING OF REHABILITATION PERSONNEL

Vocational Rehabilitation Act of 1954 as Amended

Rehabilitation training in mental retardation began in the 1950s, supported with funds from the "salaries and expenses" budget line of the Department of Health, Education, and Welfare, Office of Vocational Rehabilitation, and was one of the earliest federally supported mental retardation activities. The 1954 Amendments to the Vocational Rehabilitation Act, under Section 4 (a) (1), had supported short-term training institutes and seminars dating back as early as 1956. The purpose of these short-term training institutes, seminars, and workshops was to increase the technical proficiency of rehabilitation personnel working in this field. A major step forward oc-

curred in 1964 with the proposal to create regional centers for training. These were the mental retardation "Rehabilitation Research and Training Centers" at the Universities of Wisconsin, Texas, and Oregon.

In 1968, PL 90-391 amended Section 4 (a)(1) by specifying that a portion of this section's activity should deal with "problems related to the rehabilitation of the mentally retarded." The language of this provision was construed to not require vocational objectives for projects funded under Section 4(a)(1), but rather to authorize activities for young and severely retarded persons. The year 1973 brought a comprehensive revision of the entire Vocational Rehabilitation Act, including its training provisions. Thus, between FY 1974 and FY 1978, training was funded under Section 203 of Title II of the Rehabilitation Act of 1973. Amendments to the act in 1978 (PL

95-602) reframed Title II training provisions as Title III, Section 304. (See Table 24 for the vocational rehabilitation training authorized under the 1954 act, as amended.)

Rehabilitation training today is organized around noncategorical disciplines such as rehabilitation counseling, rehabilitation medicine, physical and occupational therapy, pros-

Table 24. Vocational rehabilitation training authorized under the 1954 Vocational Rehabilitation Act as Amended: FY 1963–1985 (dollars are in thousands)

FY	Total training funds	MR % of rehabilitants	Estimated MR expenditures
1963	$13,300	5.4	$718
1964	$16,505	6	$990
1965	$19,810	7.6	$1,506
1966	$24,800	9.3	$2,306
1967	$29,700	10.2	$3,029
1968	$31,712	10.5	$3,330
1969	$31,700	11.4	$3,614
1970	$27,700	11.8	$3,269
1971	$31,000	12.5	$3,875
1972	$26,700	11.6	$3,097
1973	$33,265	12.1	$4,025
1974	$15,507	12.6	$1,954
1975	$18,938	12.4	$2,348
1976	$22,089	12.2	$2,695
1977	$30,493	12.2	$3,720
1978	$25,000	12.4	$3,100
1979	$20,000	12.1	$2,420
1980	$30,500	11.7	$3,569
1981	$28,500	11.6	$3,306
1982	$21,675	12.4	$2,688
1983	$19,200	12	$2,304
1984	$19,200	12	$2,304
1985	$22,000	12	$2,640

Source: Total training funds exclude DD Demonstration Grants funded under Section 4 (a)(1) in FY 1972–74. They also exclude Research and Training Center funds and Hospital Improvement Project (HIP) and HIST Project funds. Data for FY 1963–72 were obtained from Braddock (1973, p. 101) and from the RSA for FY 1973–84 (H. Shay, personal communication, October 30, 1984). Data for FY 1985 are from the Handicapped Americans report (10/18/84, p. 4).

The third column of the table refers to the percentage of total clients rehabilitated in the state-federal rehabilitation program who were mentally retarded or developmentally disabled. The source of mental retardation caseload figures was the Office of the RSA Commissioner (L. Mars, personal communication). Estimates of the extent to which the rehabilitation training program has supported mental retardation activities must, unfortunately, rely on a questionable assumption, or not be made at all. The most logical assumption is that trainees involved in rehabilitation training programs in state rehabilitation agencies and universities receive assistance in rough proportion to the percentage of clients with mental retardation reported rehabilitated under the state grant program (e.g., 10% of all rehabilitants in FY 1967 were mentally retarded or developmentally disabled; therefore, 10% of training funds expended were allocated for mental retardation purposes).

The last column presents specific mental retardation training figures for FY 1963–71, identified in an examination of federal project grant descriptions completed by the RSA Division of Project Grant Administration in 1972 (Braddock, 1973, p. 101). These figures underestimate mental retardation efforts because they do not reflect the share of general noncategorical training expenditures attributable to mental retardation during the period. Data for FY 1972–74 are from the FY 1974 record of House hearings (Office of Mental Retardation Coordination [OMRC] 1974, p. 5). Data for FY 1975 are from House hearings on the FY 1977 HEW budget (OHI, 1976, p. 10). Data for 1976–79 are from FY 1980 House budget hearings (U.S. House of Representatives [House], 1979, p. 596). Data for FY 1980–81 are from FY 1981 House hearings on the HEW budget (House, 1980).

thetics-orthotics, speech pathology, and audiology. Curriculum content on mental retardation and developmental disabilities was and continues to be included within the course of study of the various disciplines. Clinical field-work experience is carried out in MR/DD facilities and agencies. In addition, training support is provided for state rehabilitation agency personnel through continuing education programs to improve professional skills in rehabilitating persons with MR/DD and other disabilities.

Unadjusted spending for mental retardation training activities increased almost every year from FY 1963 to FY 1973. The peak expenditure was $4 million in 1973; thereafter, the general trend moved downward to $2.3 million in FY 1984. The FY 1985 appropriation of $2.6 million was 15% above the 1984 figure (see Figure 45).

In real economic terms, the expenditures peaked in FY 1968–69, and fell consistently thereafter through FY 1984. A 9% increase

was budgeted for FY 1985. The FY 1985 adjusted figure, however, was only 22% of the sum budgeted 16 years earlier in FY 1969. Funding for the total program of training for vocational rehabilitation personnel parallels the trends in mental retardation training funding (see Figure 46).

TRAINING OF BIOMEDICAL AND HEALTH SERVICES PERSONNEL

National Institute of Child Health and Human Development: PL 87-838, Title IV E, Section 411

The National Institute of Child Health and Human Development was established in 1962 by PL 87-838, Title IV, Part E, which embodied one of the major recommendations of the report of the President's Panel on Mental Retardation (1962). Within the National Institutes of Health, the NICHD has primary re-

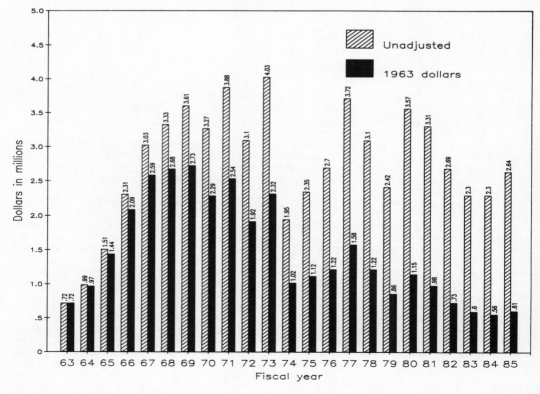

Figure 45.   Estimated mental retardation expenditures for the training of vocational rehabilitation personnel: FY 1963–85.

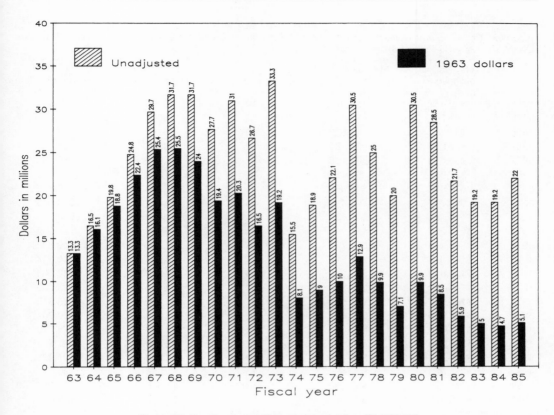

Figure 46.   Vocational rehabilitation training funding: FY 1963–85.

sponsibility for research concerned with mental retardation and developmental disabilities. This function is administratively coordinated by the institute's MR/DD branch of the Center for Research on Mothers and Children (CRMC). The MR/DD branch supports research on the biological, behavioral, and social processes that influence human development. Of primary concern are studies dealing with the etiology and prevention of mental retardation and other developmental disabilities. Other research pertaining to MR/DD prevention is also supported in the activities of other branches of the CRMC. Twelve mental retardation research centers located throughout the United States are funded by NICHD and administered by the institute's MR/DD branch. At FY 1984 House budget hearings (U.S. House of Representatives [House], 1983), the institute indicated that in FY 1982, it supported 137 extramural research grants and

contracts directly concerned with the epidemiology, etiology, diagnosis, and prevention of mental retardation and developmental disabilities. (See Table 25 for the funding patterns from FY 1964 to FY 1985.)

In unadjusted terms, support for mental retardation training rose rapidly during the first few years after the creation of the institute (see Figure 47). In FY 1969 funding dipped slightly, but resumed its steady annual increase through FY 1978, with the exception of an erratic disruption in FY 1973–74. Then, between FY 1978 and FY 1984, training support fell by 29% on an unadjusted basis from $1.9 million to $1.4 million. An increase of 32% was projected in FY 1985 spending for MR/DD training over the FY 1984 level. On an adjusted basis, annual growth was basically strong through FY 1974, but the spending level a decade later had plummeted to only 27% of the FY 1974 peak.

Table 25. National Institute of Child Health and Human Development, Public Law 87-838, Title IV, Part E as Amended; Research and Training support in Mental Retardation, Center for Mothers and Children, MR Branch ONLY: FY 1964–85 (dollars are in thousands)

FY	Total NICHD obligations	MR/DD research and training funding	% MR	MR/DD training funding	MR/DD research funding
1964	$30,462	$3,022	10	$196	$2,826
1965	$41,097	$3,281	8	$303	$2,978
1966	$53,734	$4,629	9	$744	$3,885
1967	$62,237	$6,105	10	$937	$5,168
1968	$66,830	$7,106	11	$1,077	$5,939
1969	$71,091	$8,634	12	$1,035	$7,599
1970	$76,502	$10,560	14	$1,208	$9,352
1971	$94,747	$14,490	15	$1,347	$13,143
1972	$116,498	$19,750	17	$1,474	$18,276
1973	$111,207	$19,216	17	$957	$18,259
1974	$144,146	$21,731	15	$2,109	$19,622
1975	$126,399	$22,372	18	$1,535	$20,837
1976	$135,873	$23,946	18	$1,582	$22,364
1977	$145,111	$25,370	17	$1,778	$23,592
1978	$165,817	$27,544	17	$1,927	$25,617
1979	$197,349	$30,883	16	$1,680	$29,203
1980	$208,346	$30,303	15	$1,724	$28,529
1981	$220,366	$29,497	13	$1,545	$27,952
1982	$226,172	$29,262	12	$1,278	$27,984
1983	$254,323	$32,496	13	$1,555	$30,941
1984	$275,179	$35,832	13	$1,360	$31,219
1985	$313,295	$36,921	12	$1,826	$35,095

Source: Figures were provided by the NICHD Financial Management Section (J. Zagata, Budget Analyst, personal communications, July 18, 1983, November 22, 1983, and November 21, 1984). Figures are actual obligations through 1983. FY 1984 figures are revised estimates appropriated subsequent to the enactment of the 1984 DHHS Appropriations Act. FY 1985 figures are final congressional appropriations. Research figures include only MR/DD branch funds for extramural and intramural research. In FY 1981–82, intramural research was approximately 6% of total MR/DD research expenditures at the agency.(See also Chapter 5.)

National Institute of Neurological and Communicative Disorders and Stroke: Public Health Services Act, Title IV D

The involvement of the National Institute of Neurological and Communicative Disorders and Stroke (NINCDS) in mental retardation and developmental disabilities research and training activity is of considerable historical importance. NINCDS, formerly the National Institute of Neurological Diseases and Stroke, began supporting clinical training in mental retardation in FY 1954. Through FY 1972, training activities sponsored by the institute included fellowships and institutional training grants. Cross-disciplinary training such as pe-

diatric training for neurologists and behavioral science training for pediatricians strengthened the clinical ability to identify and treat mental retardation. In 1955, the House Labor-HEW Subcommittee on Appropriations added $500,000 to the NINCDS budget request for FY 1956 and explicitly instructed it to expend these funds for mental retardation research. The subcommittee clearly intended the NINCDS to be central to the development of the national research mission in mental retardation.

The current research program supported by NINCDS is primarily concerned with disorders of early childhood. These disorders include metabolic diseases, such as Tay Sach's

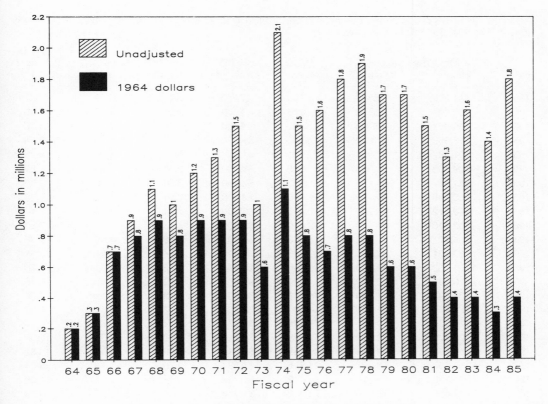

Figure 47. NICHD financial support for MR/DD training: FY 1964–85.

and phenylketonuria (PKU); cerebral palsy; birth injuries; and spina bifida. Scientific investigations funded by NINCDS also focus on a variety of basic biological, biochemical, and molecular studies of the development and function of the nervous system. These studies are designed to provide a new understanding of nervous system development and functioning. According to FY 1984 House hearings, the NINCDS was supporting 58 extramural studies on mental retardation and metabolic disorders that affect the brain and are known to cause mental retardation (House, 1983).

Support for training showed a precipitous drop in FY 1973. The amounts shown for MR/DD training activities for FY 1954–72 ranged between 25% and 36% of total NINCDS training program funding, while MR/DD related training for FY 1973–82 was between 10% and 20% of total training funding (see Table 26). According to the

NINCDS, this decrease in percentage as well as a decrease in dollars was a result of several factors (B. Matthews, personal communications, July 22, 1983, July 27, 1983, and November 15, 1984).

In 1973, the "old" training program was repealed by law when the National Research Service Award (NRSA) Act was passed. As the old training programs were phased out, the result was fewer NRSA fellowships and institutional training grants supporting clinical training, such as for pediatric neurologists. None of the current NRSA training programs of the institute is specifically or exclusively directed toward mental retardation and developmental disabilities. Training activities are, however, directed toward the development of clinical neurologists and investigators in fields associated with disorders of the nervous system. These disciplines provide the basic tools required for any serious attack on the problem

Table 26.   NINCDS research and training support for MR/DD under the Public Health Service Act, Title IV, Part D: FY 1954–85 (dollars are in thousands)

FY	Total NINCDS budget	MR/DD research & training $	MR/DD research $	MR/DD training $	% MR/DD research	% MR/DD training	% MR/DD training & research
1954	$4,500	$326	$165	$170	3.47	3.78	7.24
1955	$7,601	$575	$275	$300	3.62	3.95	7.56
1956	$9,861	$795	$335	$460	3.40	4.66	8.06
1957	$18,650	$1,590	$590	$1,000	3.16	5.36	8.53
1958	$21,387	$1,895	$695	$1,200	3.25	5.61	8.86
1959	$29,403	$2,615	$1,015	$1,600	3.45	5.44	8.89
1960	$41,487	$3,775	$1,375	$2,400	3.31	5.78	9.10
1961	$56,600	$4,160	$1,760	$2,400	3.11	4.24	7.35
1962	$70,812	$5,270	$2,270	$3,000	3.21	4.24	7.44
1963	$83,506	$6,010	$2,610	$3,400	3.13	4.07	7.20
1964	$84,471	$7,080	$2,980	$4,100	3.53	4.85	8.38
1965	$87,821	$7,600	$3,200	$4,400	3.64	5.01	8.65
1966	$101,153	$8,800	$3,700	$5,100	3.66	5.04	8.70
1967	$116,396	$10,200	$4,300	$5,900	3.69	5.07	8.76
1968	$128,633	$11,400	$4,800	$6,600	3.73	5.13	8.86
1969	$128,934	$11,000	$4,800	$6,200	3.72	4.81	8.53
1970	$106,978	$10,966	$4,795	$6,171	4.48	5.77	10.25
1971	$105,807	$12,011	$5,795	$6,216	5.48	5.87	11.35
1972	$116,590	$12,381	$6,169	$6,212	5.29	5.33	10.62
1973	$130,692	$6,322	$4,835	$1,487	3.70	1.14	4.84
1974	$121,358	$7,276	$5,412	$1,864	4.46	1.54	6.00
1975	$142,498	$5,326	$3,842	$1,484	2.70	1.04	3.74
1976	$144,446	$6,294	$5,060	$1,234	3.50	0.85	4.36
1977	$155,500	$5,289	$4,688	$601	3.01	0.39	3.40
1978	$178,438	$6,680	$5,646	$1,034	3.16	0.58	3.74
1979	$212,365	$7,815	$6,631	$1,184	3.12	0.56	3.68
1980	$241,966	$10,827	$8,536	$2,291	3.53	0.95	4.47
1981	$252,533	$10,116	$8,908	$1,208	3.53	0.48	4.01
1982	$265,901	$8,963	$8,205	$758	3.09	0.29	3.37
1983	$297,056	$7,896	$7,072	$824	2.38	0.28	2.66
1984	$335,952	$7,542	$6,635	$907	1.97	0.27	2.24
1985	$396,885	$8,890	$7,665	$1,225	1.93	0.31	2.24

Source: DHHS, NIH, NINCDS, Budget Officer (B. Matthews, personal communications, July 22, 1983, July 27, 1983, and November 15, 1984); Braddock (1973, p. 74). (The MR/DD research funding figures in Column 4 are analyzed in Chapter 5.)

of organically based MR/DD. The current NRSA program supports disciplines such as developmental neurology, speech pathology, speech perception, and audiology.

In unadjusted terms, funding for training advanced from $170,000 in FY 1954 to its peak of $6.6 million in FY 1968. The following year, it dropped by 6% to $6.2 million and leveled off through FY 1972. On an adjusted basis, funding for MR/DD training followed a nearly identical pattern. These trends are displayed in Figure 48.

As just mentioned, in 1973, with the passage of the NRSA Act, the institute's training strategy was refocused toward such areas as clinical neurology and research preparation in basic developmental neurobiology. Figure 49 presents trends in NINCDS support for train-

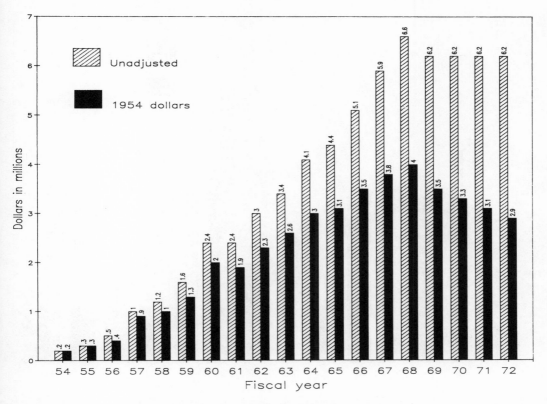

Figure 48. NINCDS funding for MR/DD training: FY 1954–72.

ing in clinical neurobiology for FY 1973–85.

As shown in Figure 49, funding for the clinical neurobiology component has ranged from a peak of $2.3 million in FY 1980 to a low of $600,000 in FY 1977. For 7 of the past 12 years, funding ranged between $1 million and $1.8 million. In real economic terms, however, NINCDS training funds have plunged dramatically since FY 1973. Estimated MR/DD training expenditures at NINCDS in 1985 were only 33% of their adjusted FY 1973 level. Meanwhile, the agency's total budget has been increasing consistently year after year. Only once in the last 30 years has the institute's budget exhibited a significant drop—that was in FY 1970. In FY 1973, impounded institute funds were released, temporarily inflating that year's actual obligations, and giving the appearance of a budget cut in FY 1974. The

institute's budget history is presented in Figure 50.

Social Security Act, Title V, Sections 511, 503, and 504

Title V, Section 516 (changed to Section 511 in 1969) of the Social Security Act as Amended authorized grants to be made for the training of health care personnel related to the provision of services to mothers and children, particularly children with mental retardation and children with multiple handicaps. The Section 511 training program had its beginnings in 1963 under PL 88-164, which authorized federal support for the construction of University Affiliated Facilities to house new training efforts. Many of the universities that applied for these construction grants were already receiving funding for clinical services to

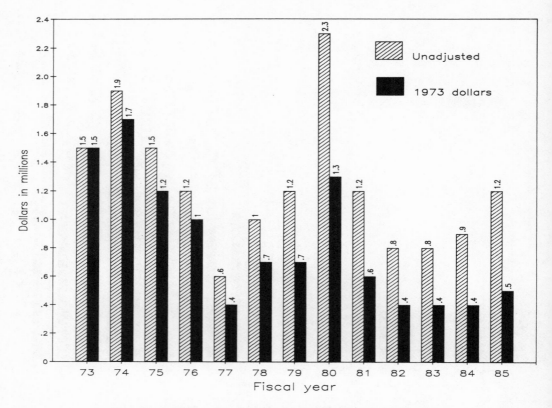

Figure 49. NINCDS funding for training in clinical neurobiology: FY 1973–85.

children with mental retardation from the HEW Maternal and Child Health (MCH) Service.

Although explicit support for UAFs was not stipulated in Section 511, UAFs received virtually all Section 511 funds for the FY 1967–71 period. In FY 1972–73, about 10% of the amounts appropriated pursuant to Section 511 were obligated for purposes other than mental retardation, such as for training nurse midwives, physician assistants, and other allied health personnel. As overall funding support for Section 511 grew, the proportion of funds allocated for purposes other than mental retardation increased at an even more rapid rate. On October 1, 1981, the consolidated Maternal and Child Health Block Grant was established under provisions of the Omnibus Budget Reconciliation Act (PL 97-35). Training and Section 511 funds were folded into the new block grant, with the requirement that

15% of the total funds expended be deployed for federally administered "special projects," which included research and training activities. Spending figures for mental retardation listed in Table 27 for FY 1982–85, were estimated by the MCH Training Office.

Much smaller sums of money also supported training activities under Sections 503 and 504 of Title V. Sections 503 and 504 training funds were "informally" deployed from MCH and Crippled Children's (CC) state formula grant funds for FY 1972–76. In FY 1977, this administrative practice was discontinued. Training activities that had been supported under Sections 503 and 504 were shifted to Section 511 support.

Section 511 support for mental retardation training activities advanced consistently from $3.9 million in FY 1967, the program's first year, to $15.1 million in FY 1972. A temporary plateau was reached during FY 1973–74

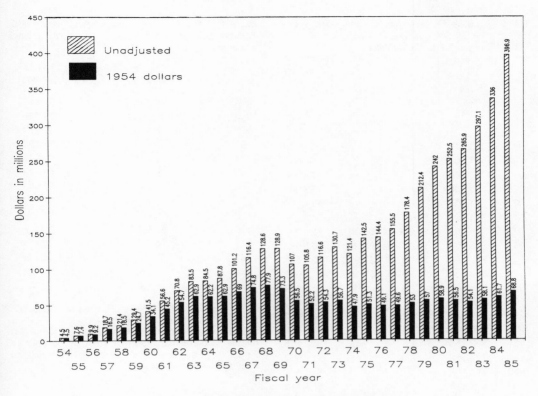

Figure 50.   NINCDS budget history (obligations): FY 1954–85.

at \$15.9 million. Funding continued to rise aggressively from FY 1975 to FY 1979, reaching a zenith at \$26.9 million. Program funding dropped marginally in FY 1980 to \$26.0 million, the first decline in the program's history. If, however, the training funds which were expended under Sections 503 and 504 during FY 1972–76 are included, the growth pattern evens out and displays steadier increases through those years.

In FY 1981, when the MCH Block Grant was authorized, the program's funding saw a rapid and unparalleled decline. Support dropped 15% in FY 1981, 21% in FY 1982, and an additional 2% in FY 1984. The FY 1985 figure was projected to be identical to the FY 1984 level.

In real economic terms, the decline was 59% between FY 1979 and FY 1985. The FY 1985 adjusted spending figure for mental retardation and developmental disabilities was approximately equivalent to funding during

the first year of the program in FY 1967. These trends are illustrated in Figure 51.

Since FY 1981, about \$2 million annually of these funds support Biochemical and Cytogenetic Laboratory training programs, located in 15 medical schools throughout the United States. Another approximately \$2 million annually goes to scattered continuing education programs predominantly focused on MR/DD. The remainder is deployed to UAFs.

Public Health Services Act, Title V, Section 303 (HIST)

Title V of the Public Health Services Act Amendments of 1956 authorized a mental health project grant program under Section 303. In FY 1964, this grant program was expanded to provide funds for the demonstration of methods of care, treatment, and rehabilitation of residents of public institutions for mentally ill and for mentally retarded persons. Hospital Improvement Project grants and

Table 27.   MR/DD training funds under the Social
Security Act, Title V, Sections 511, 503, and 504: FY
1967–85 (dollars are in thousands)

FY	MCH Sec. 511 block grant training	Sec. 503 MCH training	Sec. 504 CC training	Total MR/DD training
1967	$3,912			$3,912
1968	$7,000			$7,000
1969	$9,000			$9,000
1970	$9,000	—		$9,000
1971	$11,200	—	—	$11,200
1972	$15,100	$2,767	—	$17,867
1973	$15,900	$2,998	$1,341	$20,239
1974	$15,900	$2,767	$2,998	$21,665
1975	$17,900	$2,767	$2,998	$22,051
1976	$18,400	$1,992	$2,159	$23,665
1977	$23,400			$23,400
1978	$24,000			$24,000
1979	$26,900			$26,900
1980	$26,000			$26,000
1981	$22,156			$22,156
1982	$17,552			$17,552
1983	$17,452			$17,452
1984	$17,118			$17,118
1985	$17,118			$17,118

Source: FY 1967–71 data are from Braddock
(1973, p. 83); FY 1972–85 data are from the DHHS,
Public Health Services, Health Services Administra-
tion, Division of Maternal and Child Health, Office of
Training (J. Papai, personal communications,
November, 1983, and December 6, 1984).
   Funding levels for Sections 503 (Maternal and
Child Health; MCH) and 504 (Crippled Children; CC),
which supported training activities during FY 1972–
76, were obtained from the FY 1974 House hearings
(OHI, 1975, p. 66).
   With the initiation of the MCH Block Grant, identifying MR/DD training funding in the states became
much more difficult. FY 1981–84 figures were provided by Papai (personal communication, December
6, 1984). Figures include training at UAFs, Biochemical and Cytogenetic Laboratories, and various
other continuing education and single discipline training grants focusing on MR/DD.

Table 28.   Public Health Services Act, Section 303,
HIP and HIST Project funding: FY 1964–77 (dollars
are in thousands)

FY	HIP MR funding	HIST MR funding
1964	$2,153	$1,119
1965	$4,305	$1,840
1966	$6,630	$2,279
1967	$6,689	$2,189
1968	$6,135	$2,386
1969	$6,551	$2,547
1970	$6,096	$2,370
1971	$5,976	$2,324
1972	$4,680	$1,820
1973	$2,986	$496
1974	$4,477	$774
1975	$5,997	$449
1976	$0	$394
1977	$0	$146

Source: Data for FY 1964–72 are from Braddock
(1973, p. 77); data for FY 1973–74 are from FY 1975
House appropriations hearings (Office of Mental Retardation Coordination [OMRC], 1974, p. 61); data for
FY 1975–77 are from FY 1977 House appropriations
hearings (OHI, 1976, p. 8).

grants for Hospital In-Service Training were
supported in state-operated MR/DD residential facilities between 1964 and 1977.
   From FY 1964 to FY 1967, the demonstration and training programs were administered
by the Division of Mental Health Services of
the National Institute of Mental Health.

Thereafter, following the FY 1967 Department of Health, Education, and Welfare reorganization, mental retardation components
of both the HIP and HIST Programs were
transferred to the newly established Division
of Mental Retardation in the new Social and
Rehabilitation Service (SRS). HIP grants had
a ceiling of $100,000 per institution; HIST, a
ceiling of $25,000. In FY 1973, there were
projects operating in 111 state mental retardation institutions.
   Four general types of training were supported by HIST grants: 1) initial on-the-job
training for employees; 2) refresher, continuing, and other special job-related training;
3) continuing education for professional staff
on new developments in the field; and 4) special "train-the-trainer" training for staff with
in-service training responsibilities. Table 28
shows the history of HIP and HIST funding
for MR/DD projects. The expenditure trends
of the two programs are further illustrated in
Figure 52.

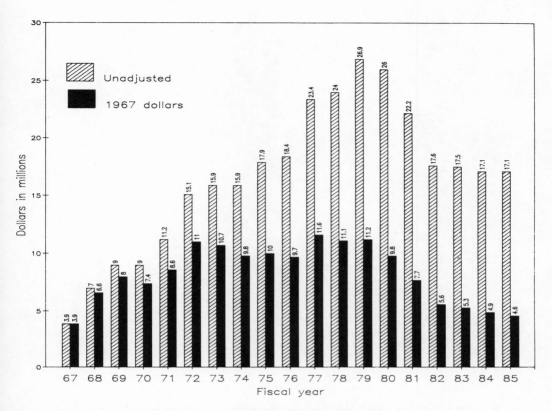

Figure 51. MR/DD training support under Section 511 and the MCH Block Grant Program: FY 1967–85.

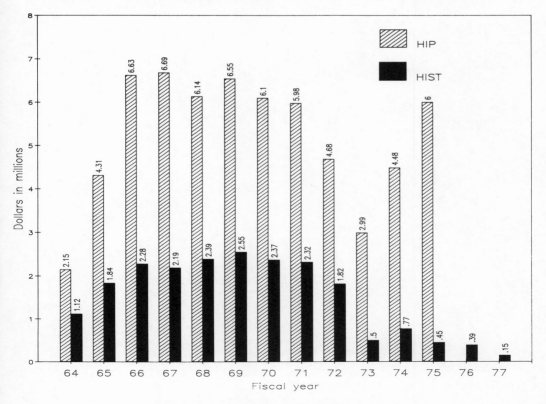

Figure 52. Funding history of HIP and HIST: FY 1964–77.

Chapter 5

Research Programs

IN A GENERAL sense, federal government research on MR/DD began with the U.S. Census Bureau's efforts in the 1840 decennial census to enumerate the number of persons with mental retardation living in the United States. After the turn of the century, the U.S. Children's Bureau, created by statute in 1912 as a component of the U.S. Department of Labor, financed the first three noncensus demographic studies. *Mental Defectives in the District of Columbia* (1915); *A Social Study of Mental Defectives in New Castle County, Delaware* (Lundberg, 1917); and *Mental Defect in a Rural County* (Treadway & Lundberg, 1919) were the new bureau's 13th, 24th, and 48th publications, respectively. In 1923, the bureau published a study of the employment history of minors who had been pupils in special classes (U.S. Children's Bureau, 1964).

In the decades that followed, the bureau conducted occasional sociological and demographic studies. At the same time, the U.S. Office of Education, under the leadership of Else Martin and Romaine Mackie, published several national surveys between 1920 and 1965 on services provided to exceptional children in the public schools (Mackie, 1969). Boggs (1971) noted that these surveys helped document the regression in public services to persons with mental retardation or developmental disabilities brought on by the Great Depression and World War II.

MR/DD biomedical research received its first major impetus in 1950, with the formation of the National Association for Retarded Citizens (NARC; Boggs, 1971). The first NARC constitution stipulated research on pre-vention and amelioration of mental retardation as an important national priority. A scientific advisory board was appointed to address these issues, the result of which was a recommendation that a comprehensive study be completed on the status of biomedical research on mental retardation. Such a study, led by Richard Masland (Masland, Sarason, & Gladwin, 1958), was initiated in 1954 with foundation and, later, National Institute of Neurological Diseases and Blindness (NINDB) assistance. Also during the early 1950s, the federal government began supporting the country's first demonstration projects aimed at providing rehabilitation services to clients with mental retardation. The Vocational Rehabilitation Act Amendments of 1954 then provided an effective legislative vehicle, through Section 4 (a)(1), to expand these demonstrations to many parts of the country.

It was the February, 1955, Fogarty subcommittee hearings on FY 1956 appropriations for the Department of Health, Education, and Welfare (DHEW), however, that provided the first major public stimulus for increased research funding. The subcommittee added $500,000 and $250,000 to the budget requests of the NINDB and National Institute of Mental Health (NIMH), respectively, to be exclusively devoted to mental retardation research. The Office of Education, which had been instructed in 1955 to return to the budget hearings 1 year later with a proposed mental retardation program plan, initiated educational studies in mental retardation under the auspices of the Cooperative Research Act (PL 83-531) in FY 1960.

In the early years, mental retardation research support increased annually at the federal level. Funds budgeted advanced from $1.4 million in FY 1956 to $47.1 million in FY 1971, as illustrated in Figure 53. After FY 1971, however, research was no longer the budget priority it had been. Cuts in overall federal mental retardation research funding were sustained in FY 1972, FY 1973, FY 1975, FY 1976, FY 1981, FY 1982, and FY 1984. The rate of budget growth also slowed considerably. Whereas the unadjusted growth of mental retardation research support had averaged 20% annually between FY 1963 and FY 1972, growth averaged only 1.1% for the FY 1973–82 period on a yearly basis. In FY 1984, MR/DD research spending fell fractionally to $57.8 million. The FY 1985 spending figure was $64.56 million, an increase of 12% over the previous year's level. The increase is primarily attributable to rising fund-

ing for the National Institute of Child Health and Human Development (NICHD), National Institute of Neurological and Communicative Disorders and Stroke (NINCDS), and National Institute of Allergy and Infectious Diseases (NIAID).

Adjusting research funding trends for the impact of inflation reveals rapid growth from FY 1954 to FY 1972, although the rate of that positive growth slowed to 3% per annum during FY 1966–70. There was a 36% real dollar expansion in research funding between FY 1965 and FY 1966 with the establishment and funding of the NICHD, the Rehabilitation Research and Training Centers, and the special education research authority authorized under Title III of PL 88-164. Funding regressed, however, almost every year between FY 1971 and FY 1984. The average rate of decline was 5.5% annually over this 12-year span. The total drop in research spending was 54%. Real

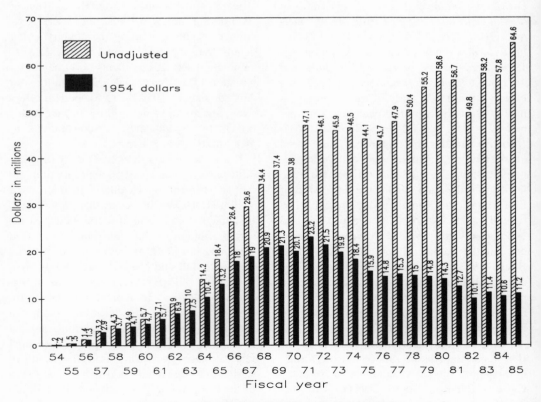

Figure 53.   Federal funding of MR/DD research: FY 1954–85.

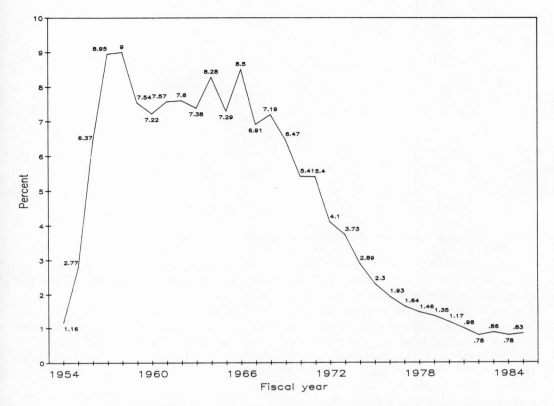

Figure 54.   Federal MR/DD research expenditures as a percentage of total federal MR/DD expenditures: FY 1954–85.

research spending increased in FY 1985 by 5.7% over the FY 1984 figure.

Spending for mental retardation and developmental disabilities research, as a percentage of total federal MR/DD expenditures, has declined over the years (see Figure 54). In the field's developing years, MR/DD research made up a very large part of the federal mission. From FY 1956 to FY 1971, in fact, the percentage ranged between 9% and 5.4% of total federal government MR/DD expenditures. Since FY 1972, and the ensuing period of explosive growth in federal services and income maintenance expenditures, the MR/DD research share has plunged to less than 1% of total MR/DD expenditures. As the federal government has expended more and more funds on MR/DD activities, it has expended proportionately less and less resources on research and development activities relevant to that mission. Figure 55 depicts antici-

pated federal expenditures for MR/DD research in FY 1985; the data were based on enacted FY 1985 appropriations.

As with funding for personnel training, the federal government has been financing MR/DD research for more than 30 years. Also, as with personnel training, federal research activity is divisible into 3 general categories of activity: 1) educational research; 2) vocational rehabilitation research; and 3) biomedical, behavioral, and health services research. The rest of this chapter describes federal expenditures for each program under the three broad research categories.

EDUCATION RESEARCH

Title VI, Part E, PL 91-230: EHA Special Education Research

Research in special education was initiated during FY 1964 with the appropriation of

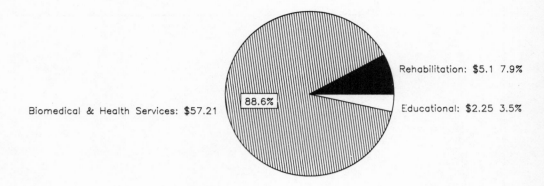

Rehabilitation: $5.1 7.9%

Biomedical & Health Services: $57.21   88.6%

Educational: $2.25 3.5%

Total: $64.56 Million

Figure 55.   Federal spending for MR/DD research: FY 1985. (Dollars are in millions.)

$1 million authorized under Title III, Section 302 of PL 88-164, the Mental Retardation Facilities and Community Mental Health Centers Construction Act. This authorization has been continued and the scope and flexibility of the program have been expanded over the years. The program, now the Research Projects Branch of the Office of Special Education (OSE), U.S. Department of Education, supports research and related activities that show promise of leading to improvement in educational programs for children with handicaps. Support is available for research, dissemination, demonstration, curriculum, and media activities (Table 29 is restricted to research funding only).

Many of the special education research projects funded in the 1960s were primarily focused on mental retardation issues. However, in the 1970s, the trend toward noncategorical research was strong. Now, it seems that specific fiscal support for mental retardation activities has diminished. Max Mueller, who headed this branch for many years, noted in an interview that the research program has virtually stopped receiving proposals for educable mentally retarded (EMR) research, but it continues to receive similar proposals under the rubric of "mildly handicapped" (personal communication, November 14, 1983). It is inappropriate to conclude that simply because projects are being funded

under noncategorical auspices that they do not bear an important relation to mental retardation issues.

The impact of the OSE Research Projects Branch activities on the field of mental retardation is illustrated in the following quotation from FY 1977 House hearings on the HEW budget:

As of the end of 1974, supported projects have resulted in the distribution of over 500 project reports relating to education of the mentally retarded through the Educational Resources Information Center (ERIC) system, and at least an equal number of publications in professional journals. In addition, validated curriculum materials designed specifically for mentally retarded persons have been developed and are now available in the area of social learning, arithmetic, science, physical education, and self-help skills. (Office for Handicapped Individuals [OHI], 1976, p. 26)

Special Education Instructional Materials Centers and Regional Resource Centers for handicapped children and youth actually began as development and demonstration projects supported through the research program. They currently exist in modified form and provide technical support services for teachers and clinicians working with mentally retarded and other handicapped children and youth (OH], 1976 p. 26).

In unadjusted terms, funding for special education research in mental retardation in-

Table 29. Special education research funding history: FY 1964–85 (dollars are in thousands)

FY	Total research funding	MR Research funding	No. of MR projects
1964	$1,000	$238	9
1965	$2,000	$521	14
1966	$5,994	$1,110	39
1967	$8,049	$1,084	32
1968	$10,791	$1,608	31
1969	$13,622	$1,493	27
1970	$16,000	$1,602	16
1971	$15,000	$4,413	10
1972	$15,455	$2,204	14
1973	$15,455	$3,020	27
1974	$14,438	$2,599	18
1975	$9,664	$2,706	28
1976	$20,933	$3,768	18
1977	$10,894	$3,523	28
1978	$20,000	$2,009	18
1979	$20,000	$1,530	25
1980	$20,000	$1,469	29
1981	$15,000	$1,035	18
1982	$10,800	$413	9
1983	$12,000	$2,250	25
1984	$15,000	$2,250	25
1985	$16,000	$2,250	24

Source: For FY 1964–1976, all mental retardation data are from FY 1979 House hearings (U.S. House of Representatives, 1978, p. 1177) except for FY 1969 data, which were revised as a result of discussions with the former director of the Office of Special Education Research (M. Mueller, personal communication, November 14, 1983). Data for FY 1977–82 were also provided by the OSE (M. Mueller personal communication, November 14, 1983). FY 1983–85 data were also provided by the OSE (J. Hamilton, personal communications, November 14, 1983, and November 19, 1984).

All mental retardation estimates in the table stem from actual inspection of approved project grant documents and include only those research projects "exclusively or substantially" focused on mental retardation. (Demonstrations are excluded). The figures include estimates for cross-categorical or multiple research projects in which mental retardation is the major designated focus. For example, FY 1983–84 mental retardation figures in the table reflect support for "Severely or Profoundly Handicapped" projects in which MR/DD children or youth with mental retardation are the primary targets of the research thrust.

creased dramatically from $238,000 in FY 1964 to $1.608 million in FY 1968, where it remained through FY 1970. After an atypical large increase in FY 1971, a general trend of growth continued until FY 1976 when funding reached $3.768 million. Mental retardation activities funding experienced a dramatic decrease between FY 1976 and FY 1982, plummeting to $413,000 in FY 1982. After recovering to $2.25 million in FY 1983, funding has remained at that level, which is below the funding level of a decade earlier (see Figure 56).

In real economic terms, the impact of inflation has dramatically eroded available funding in recent years. Funding for mental retardation research increased almost every year from FY 1964 to FY 1971, when it peaked in real economic terms at $3 million. By FY 1977, however, it had been cut to half its FY 1971 level. In real economic terms, expenditures projected for mental retardation research in FY 1985 were only 17% of such spending in FY 1971.

The decline of purchasing power in special education funding for mental retardation research has been accompanied by the general atrophy of the total program of federal special education research support. The entire research program authorized under Title VI, Part E of PL 91-230 as amended has been poorly funded since FY 1970, even in unadjusted terms. That year the program was funded at a level of $16 million. This figure was not exceeded or even equaled until FY 1976. Funding reached a plateau of $20 million per year during FY 1978–80, but it fell to between $15 million and $10.8 million for FY 1981–84. In FY 1985, the appropriation was increased by 6.7% to $16 million. The program has been fiscally neglected for so long, however, that the FY 1985 appropriation in real economic terms was only a third of the total research spending in FY 1970. These trends are depicted in Figure 57.

The percentage of total special education research funding devoted to mental retardation projects, as illustrated in Figure 58, has

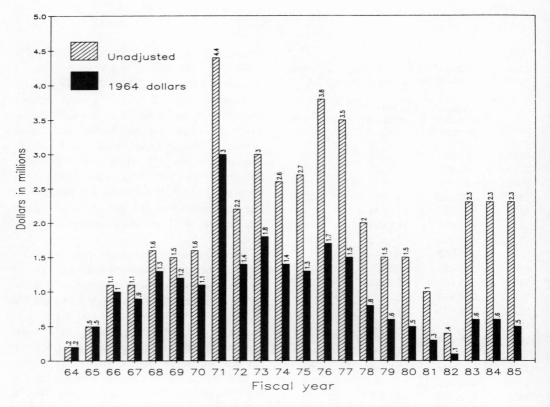

Figure 56.   Special education research funding for mental retardation activities: FY 1964–85.

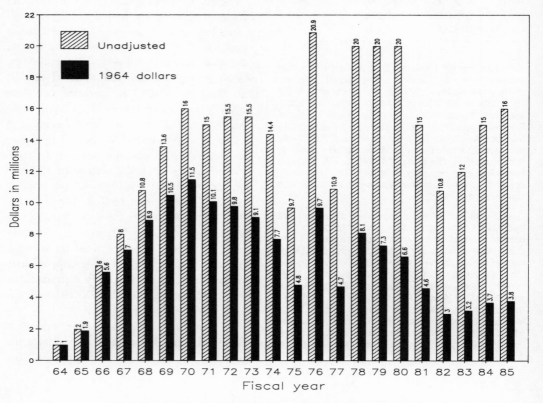

Figure 57.   Total special education research funding: FY 1964–85.

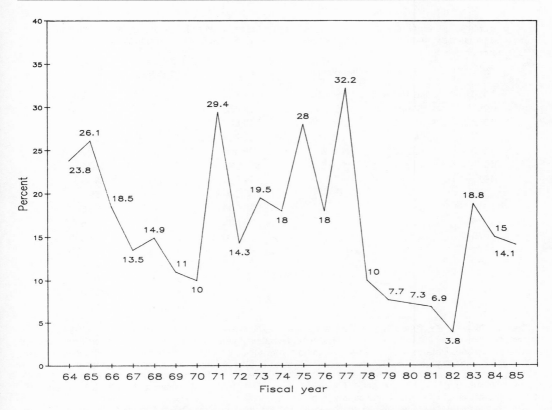

Figure 58.   Percentage of special education research projects in mental retardation: FY 1964–85.

ranged between 3.8% and 32.2%. During the 21-year history of the program, between 1964 and 1985, a total of 484 projects were funded exclusively for or substantially focused on mental retardation. The annual range was from 39 projects in FY 1966, to 9 in FY 1982.

ESEA as Amended, Titles III and IV

Title III of PL 89-750, the Elementary and Secondary Education Act (ESEA) Amendments of 1966, consolidated several educational programs for educational innovation and for the development of special services. The 1967 amendments to the ESEA, PL 90-247, required states to spend at least 15% of their Title III funds for special programs and projects pertaining to handicapped children. Federal support for Title III was recast as Title IV, Part C, of PL 95-561, the ESEA Amendments of 1978. The new act retained the 15% set-aside for education projects for children with handicaps.

In a review of expenditures under Title III of the act, Braddock (1973, pp. 60–62) examined project titles and descriptions of 182 "handicapped" Title III projects and found only 11 that dealt solely with children with mental retardation. Most of the projects included children with mental retardation among the general population served; however, the Bureau of Elementary and Secondary Education's Consolidated Program Information Report for FY 1968 (Braddock, 1973) cited categorical data indicating that children with mental retardation constituted 52.7% of the handicapped children participating in Title III that year. In 1981, the Education Consolidation and Improvement Act eliminated the earmarking for handicapped projects.

Funding for Title III and Title IV, Part C was made available for "innovative" retardation demonstration activities between FY 1966 and FY 1981 (see Table 30). During this period, funding for special activities for pupils

Table 30.   Elementary and Secondary Education Act as Amended, Title III and Title IV, Part C
estimated expenditures for mental retardation projects: FY 1966–81 (dollars are in thousands)

FY	Total Title III	All handicapped	Title III MR (est.)	Title IV C MR (est.)	Total MR (est.)
1966	$46,128	$5,352	$2,821		$2,821
1967	$162,397	$7,115	$3,750		$3,750
1968	$181,956	$12,587	$8,633		$8,633
1969	$164,767	$15,000	$7,905		$7,905
1970	$116,393	$15,870	$8,363		$8,363
1971	$143,371	$19,675	$10,369		$10,369
1972			$4,900		$4,900
1973			$8,200	—	$8,200
1974			$5,800	—	$5,800
1975			$5,800	—	$5,800
1976			$2,900	$1,555	$4,455
1977			—	$6,165	$6,165
1978			—	$6,610	$6,610
1979				$6,610	$6,610
1980				$6,610	$6,610
1981				$6,610	$6,610

Source: Data for FY 1966–71 are from Braddock (1973, p. 61); they are predicated on a 1968 program information report, which indicated that 52% of participating handicapped children in Title III projects were mentally retarded. Data for FY 1972 were obtained from Office of Mental Retardation Coordination (OMRC; 1973, p. 63). Hearings for FY 1975 contained 1973 data (Office of Mental Retardation Coordination [OMRC], 1974, p. 60). Hearings for FY 1976 presented FY 1974 figures (Office for Handicapped Individuals [OHI], 1975, p. 65). Hearings for FY 1977 presented FY 1976 figures (OHI 1976, p. 7). Hearings for FY 1978 reported FY 1977–78 estimates (Office for Handicapped Individuals [OHI], 1977, p. 268).

No HEW administrative records or testimony indicating the funds expended for handicapped children research under Title IV, Part C in FY 1979–81 could be found. Harry Phillips, director of congressional relations for the U.S. Department of Education, however, indicated in an interview that expenditures for handicapped children programs under Title IV C continued to be made during this period (personal communication, November, 1984). According to Phillips, Title IV C obligations for FY 1979–81 approximated the levels of expenditures in FY 1978. These figures were included in the table.

with mental retardation ranged from $2.8 million in FY 1966, to a high point of $10.4 million in FY 1971. Funding leveled off at $6.6 million until it was terminated in FY 1981, as illustrated in Figure 59.

National Defense Education Act of 1958 (PL 85-864) Media Research and Cooperative Research Act (PL 83-531)

The primary sources of federal financial support for educational research in the field of mental retardation during FY 1955–63 were PL 83-531 and PL 85-864. The point of initiation was in 1955 at FY 1956 budget hearings of the House HEW Appropriations Subcommittee. Although the committee did not earmark specific educational dollars during the hearings that year, it directed the Office of

Education to present a program at the budget hearings for the following year.

In 1956, at hearings on the FY 1957 Office of Education budget presented to the subcommittee, $675,000 for mental retardation research support was included pursuant to the enacted but as yet unfunded Cooperative Research Act. The Fogarty Committee approved these expenditures and during the first 18 months of the Cooperative Research Act Program nearly half of the 100 research projects funded dealt with mental retardation (Braddock, 1973, p. 128).

In FY 1959, small amounts of funds began to be spent on media research under the auspices of the newly enacted National Defense Education Act (NDEA) of 1958. Under Title VII, Section 701, the commissioner of educa-

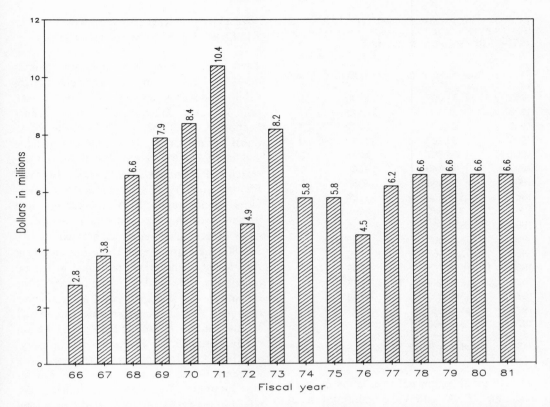

Figure 59.   Estimated mental retardation spending under Title III and Title IV, Part C of the Elementary and Secondary Education Act as Amended: FY 1966–81.

tion was authorized to make grants and contracts to promote research and development and evaluation in the presentation of academic subject matter through "television, radio, motion pictures, printed and published materials, and related communication media which may prove of value to state or local educational agencies and to institutions of higher education." Section 731 of the NDEA also empowered the commissioner to disseminate information on new educational media.

Although mental retardation funds expended under both acts are small by today's standards, these authorities permitted a significant policy departure at the federal level, and signalled greater national attention to the problem of mental retardation. Total general research support through FY 1962 under the Cooperative Research Act Program for all projects was $24.5 million. About 11.4% or

over $4.8 million was made available for research on problems in the field of mental retardation (see Table 31). Out of a total of 663 projects recommended by the commissioner of education to the Cooperative Research Advisory Committee since the beginning of the program, 77 or approximately 17% were concerned with the educational problems of individuals with mental retardation. These 77 projects were in the following research areas: cognitive processes, communication, counseling and guidance, education and training, identification and survey, and learning and measurement. There was a total of $15 million allocated under Title VII of the National Defense Education Act between FY 1959 and FY 1963, $223,000 of which was spent on mental retardation media research (U.S. House of Representatives [House], 1963, pp. 51–54) (see Table 32). During FY 1959–68, $549,000

Table 31. Cooperative Research Act as Amended (PL 83-531) mental retardation obligations: FY 1957–73 (dollars are in thousands)

FY	Total obligations	MR obligations	% MR
1957	$1,000	$648	65
1958	$2,300	$1,171	51
1959	$2,670	$972	36
1960	$3,200	$652	20
1961	$3,357	$346	10
1962	$4,640	$266	6
1963	$6,985	$367	5
1964	$11,500	$186	1.6
1965	$15,840	$190	1.2
1966	$70,000	$95	.1
1967	$70,000	$45	
1968	$66,467	$10	
1969	$94,796	$39	
1970	$92,394	$83	
1971	$88,632	$18	
1972	$110,850		
1973	$74,900		

Source: Braddock (1973, p. 127).

was obligated for mental retardation research under the NDEA, Title VII program. Financial support for Cooperative Research Projects and National Defense Education Act Media Research was terminated in FY 1972 and FY 1968, respectively. The expenditure trends for these two programs are illustrated in Figure 60.

Table 32. National Defense Education Act of 1958 (PL 85-864), Title VII Educational Media Research, mental retardation obligations: FY 1959–69 (dollars are in thousands)

FY	Total obligations	MR obligations	% MR
1959	$1,600	$9	.1
1960	$3,070	$48	1.6
1961	$4,730	$63	1.3
1962	$4,755	$82	1.7
1963	$5,000	$80	1.6
1964	$5,000	$83	1.7
1965	$4,963	$148	3.0
1966	$3,850	$26	.7
1967	$4,370	$10	.2
1968	$3,720	$0	0
1969	—	—	—

Source: Braddock (1973, p. 129).

VOCATIONAL REHABILITATION RESEARCH AND DEMONSTRATION

There are several individual program elements that have made up the federal vocational rehabilitation (VR) research mission over the past 30 years. They include support under Sections 4 (a)(1) and 4 (a)2(A) of the Vocational Rehabilitation Act of 1954 as Amended and the Mental Retardation Rehabilitation Research and Training Center Program. Between FY 1961 and FY 1977, the Rehabilitation Services Administration (RSA) also administered various research grants under the Foreign Currency Research Program authorized by PL 83-480, the Agricultural Trade Development Act. Many of the grants pertained to mental retardation. (See Table 33 for a history of the funding in the aforementioned areas.) Three relevant "special demonstration programs" are also authorized for: 1) Services to the Severely Disabled, 2) Projects with Industry, and 3) Special Recreational Activities.

Trends in research and demonstration funding pertaining to mental retardation are depicted in Figure 61. In unadjusted terms, total mental retardation rehabilitation research and demonstration activities rose from $65,000 in FY 1955 to a level of $4.01 million in FY 1966, then declined for the next 5 fiscal years. In 1968, Congress enacted a law—PL 90-391—extending Section 4(a)(1) funding to special projects for severely handicapped research and demonstrations not tied to tradiional vocational objectives. The special provision was unfunded for 2 years, but its fiscal consequences brought substantially higher mental retardation spending during FY 1972–74 (OMRC, 1974, p. 65). Mental retardation expenditures for FY 1975–76 plummeted to $1.7 million and ranged between $2 and $3 million during FY 1977–85, as depicted in Figure 62. Adjusting for the impact of inflation, total funding for rehabilitation research and demonstration activities in mental retardation surged during the 1960s and early 1970s, but has substantially declined since then. The FY 1985 adjusted level of funding is below the FY 1977 level.

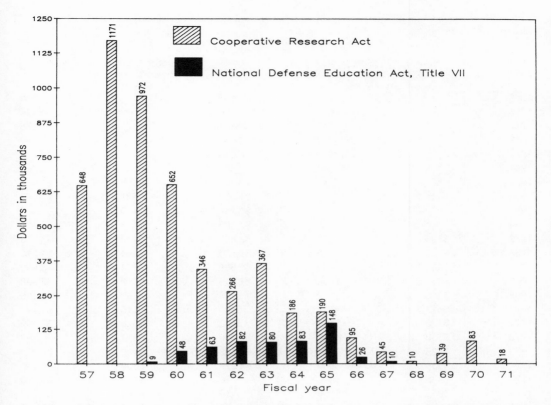

Figure 60.   Educational research supported under the Cooperative Research Act and the National Defense Education Act, Title VII: FY 1957–71.

Section 4(a)(1) and Section 202(b): Research and Training Centers

The 1954 Vocational Rehabilitation Act Amendments initiated, through Section 4(a)(1), a program of rehabilitation research, demonstration, and training. In FY 1965, mental retardation Research and Training Centers at the University of Texas at Austin and the University of Wisconsin at Madison were added to the Research and Training Center Program of the HEW Vocational Rehabilitation Administration. A third center was opened at the University of Oregon in Eugene, and the project at the University of Texas was later relocated to Texas Tech University.

The purpose of the Research and Training Centers is to conduct multidisciplinary programs of research on the major psychosocial, vocational, and personal adjustment problems

of persons with mental retardation. The Research and Training Centers' primary training responsibility has been the dissemination of research results through consultations and technical assistance, seminars, workshops, courses of study, conferences, and demonstrations that are designed to enhance the skills of students, professionals, paraprofessionals, consumers, and all other personnel involved in the rehabilitation process. In FY 1982, the Texas Tech Research and Training Center was dropped as a Research and Training Center and Virginia Commonwealth University was added in the area of the employment of handicapped persons. In 1985, Syracuse University was awarded funds to operate a new Research and Training Center on Community Integration.

Section 4(a)(1) was reframed in the Rehabilitation Act of 1973 as Title II, Section 202(b). At that time, the "other research"

Table 33.   Vocational rehabilitation research and demonstration funding in mental retardation: FY 1955–85
(dollars are in thousands)

FY	Sec. 204(a)(1) and Sec. 202(b)	Sec. 204(a)(2)(A) and Sec. 202(a)	Sec. 4(a)(1) "other research"	Foreign Currency Research Program	Total MR research
1955		$16	$49		$65
1956		$47	$97		$144
1957		$247	$131		$378
1958		$0	$448		$448
1959		$0	$524		$524
1960		$0	$862		$862
1961		$0	$927	$98	$1,025
1962		$0	$1,057	$21	$1,078
1963		$0	$1,148	$59	$1,207
1964		$0	$2,286	$138	$2,424
1965	$200	$0	$3,090	$119	$3,409
1966	$300	$86	$3,133	$494	$4,013
1967	$450	$419	$2,566	$154	$3,589
1968	$650	$450	$1,516	$382	$2,998
1969	$650	$108	$984	$393	$2,135
1970	$617	$108	$880	$16	$1,621
1971	$725	$507	$502	$528	$2,262
1972	$750	$1,230	$3,910	$317	$6,207
1973	$825	$750	$3,542	$400	$5,517
1974	$935	$800	$4,225	$300	$6,260
1975	$935	$650	$0	$125	$1,710
1976	$935	$669	$0	$100	$1,704
1977	$1,350	$1,657	$0	$100	$3,107
1978	$1,475	$1,500	$0	$0	$2,975
1979	$1,483	$1,500	$0	$0	$2,983
1980	$1,833	$1,500	$0	$0	$3,333
1981	$1,703	$200	$0	$0	$1,903
1982	$1,862	$200	$0	$0	$2,062
1983	$1,401	$487	$0	$0	$1,888
1984	$1,401	$919	$0	$0	$2,320
1985	$1,401	$389	$0	$0	$1,790

Source: Data in column two (Secs. 204[a][1] and 202[b]) are from the U.S. Department of Education, National Institute of Handicapped Research, administrative records (K. Little, program analyst, personal communications, July 21, 1983, November 16, 1983, and November 21, 1984). Column three data (Secs. 204[a][2][A] and 202[a]) refer to "Rehabilitation Research and Demonstration" in mental retardation. In the early years, this authority supported the "expansion" activities designed to accelerate services to the mentally retarded target population. Column three data for FY 1955–71 are from Braddock (1973, p. 96). FY 1973–74 data are from FY 1975 House hearings (Office of Mental Retardation Coordination [OMRC], 1973, p. 62); data for FY 1975–76 are from FY 1977 House hearings, (OHI, 1976, p. 9); FY 1976–80 data are from FY 1978 House hearings (OHI, 1977); FY 1981–85 data are from NIHR (K. Little, personal communications, November 20, 1983, and November 21, 1984).

Column four data refer only to Research and Demonstration activities funded under Section 4 (a)(1), and it excludes Research and Training Centers' core support. The centers, in the initial 10 years of operation from FY 1965 to FY 1974, had been funded through the Section 4 (a)(1) legislative authority until the Rehabilitation Act of 1973 reframed Research and Training Center support under a new Title II, Section 202 (b). Data for FY 1955–71 in column three are from Braddock (1973, p. 101); data for FY 1972–74 are from FY 1974 House Appropriations Hearings (OMRC, 1973, p. 65).

Column five presents data on funding under the Agricultural Trade Development Act of 1954 as Amended, also known as the Foreign Currency Research Program. These funds were appropriated as a part of the U.S. Department of Agriculture's budget, and routinely transferred to RSA for research expenditure. Data for FY 1961–73 are from Braddock (1973, p. 92). Data for FY 1974, FY 1975–76, and FY 1977 are from OMRC, (1973, p. 62); OHI (1976, p. 9); and the OHI (1977), respectively.

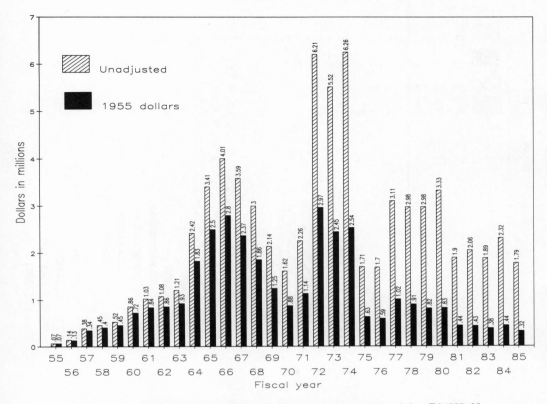

Figure 61. Rehabilitation research and demonstration funding in mental retardation: FY 1955–85.

funded by Section 4(a)(1) (see Table 33, column 4) was terminated. The act also created the National Institute of Handicapped Research to administer the rehabilitation research program.

Section 4 (a)(2)(A) and Section 202 (a): Rehabilitation Research and Demonstration

The 1954 amendments had authorized another project grant program for supporting research and demonstration activity in addition to Section 4 (a)(1). Section 4 (a)(2)(A) authorized state agencies and public or other nonprofit organizations to pay part of the cost of expanding vocational rehabilitation services and initiating special programs "holding promise of substantially increasing the number of persons rehabilitated." The House appropriations hearings record in 1963 (House, 1963 p. 57) emphasized the extensive degree to which this project grant authority was used to expand services to individuals with mental retardation.

In July, 1957, the Vocational Rehabilitation Administration (VRA) began a program of demonstration projects to accelerate services to severely disabled persons, and to provide for prompt and widespread application of knowledge and experience acquired in the VRA Research Grant Program. A total of 38 demonstration projects were approved between FY 1957 and FY 1963. Braddock (1973, p. 98) was able to identify 41 mental retardation projects in FY 1955–57, although he was not able to identify any funding for mental retardation activity under Section 4 (a)(2)(A) after 1957. With the passage of the Rehabilitation Act of 1973, Title II, Section 202 (a) reframed Section 4 (a)(2)(A) and authorized research and demonstration activities.

Foreign Currency Research Program

The Agricultural Trade Development Act of 1954 (PL 83-480) as Amended, authorized support for international research and demon-

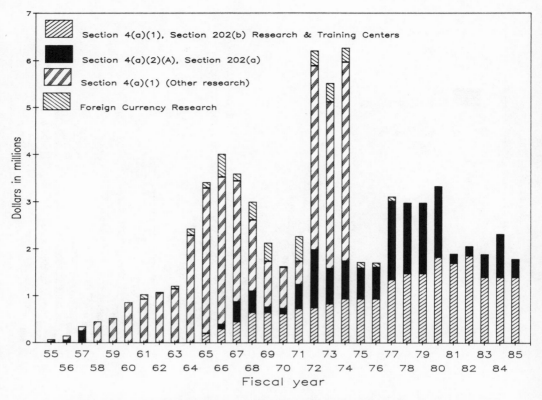

Figure 62. MR/DD rehabilitation research and demonstration funding by program element: FY 1955–85.

stration projects with U.S.-owned foreign currencies accumulated primarily from the sale of agricultural products in "excess currency countries" designated by the U.S. Treasury Department. Thirty-nine projects specifically relating to mental retardation research were identified in Braddock's inspection of project titles and descriptions for all foreign currency projects (1973, p. 94).

Between FY 1961 and FY 1977, the Foreign Currency Research Program sponsored several research projects per year dealing with the vocational rehabilitation problems of persons with mental retardation. House appropriations hearings testimony on the FY 1978 HEW budget (Office for Handicapped Individuals [OHI], 1977), for example, indicated that in FY 1977, five projects were being supported in Israel, Poland, Tanzania, and Egypt. Three new projects were proposed for FY 1978; however, the author was unable to determine if these funds were actually expended.

PL 93-112, Section 311: Severely Disabled Projects and Demonstrations
Section 311 of the Rehabilitation Act of 1973 authorized grants to states and other public and nonprofit organizations for special demonstration projects relating to serving severely handicapped persons, especially persons with spinal cord injuries, deaf-blind individuals, regardless of their rehabilitation potential. The number of projects focusing exclusively or substantially on MR/DD individuals has varied from between one and five projects during FY 1979–84. Examples of MR/DD projects include: a transitional school-work program for 58 students with severe mental retardation, a university-based community employment training project for persons with severe mental retardation, training of adults with severe mental retardation for food service work placements, and training of individuals with severe MR/DD for sheltered workshop placement. (See Table 34 for the funding history.)

Table 34. Funding history of Sections 311, 621, and 316: FY 1974–85 (dollars are in thousands)

FY	Severely Disabled: Sec. 311		Projects with Industry: Sec. 62		Special Recreation: Sec. 316	
	Total	MR/DD	Total	MR/DD	Total	MR/DD
1974	$1,000					
1975	$1,295					
1976	$2,700					
1977	$4,099					
1978	$7,048			$475		
1979	$7,048	$108		$475		
1980	$9,568	$265		$475		
1981	$9,765	$433		$475	$2,000	$490
1982	$8,855	$357	$7,510	$1,497	$1,884	$260
1983	$11,259	$705	$8,000	$2,029	$2,000	$281
1984	$11,200	$705	$13,000	$2,029	$2,000	$169
1985	$14,600	$709	$14,400	$2,429	$2,100	$169

Source: Severely Disabled Projects and Demonstrations data are from RSA, Office of Developmental Programs, (R. Gilmore, project officer, personal communications, November 9, 1983, and November 20, 1984). MR/DD data were identified from Gilmore's review of project grant titles and descriptions. Projects with Industry data are from the same source as above except for FY 1984–85 data (W. Devins, Projects with Industry project officer, personal communications, November 9, 1983, and November 20, 1984). Special Recreation data are also from Gilmore, as above, except for FY 1984–85 data (F. Caracciolo, Special Recreation Program project officer, personal communications, November 9, 1983, November 16, 1983, and November 19, 1984.)

MR/DD figures were ascertained from the author's examination of project titles and descriptions. The criterion employed in determining whether a project was to be included in the author's analysis was whether or not it was exclusively or substantially concerned with an MR/DD clientele.

PL 93-112, Section 621: Projects with Industry

Section 621 authorizes the federal government to enter into agreements with individual employers to establish jointly financed projects, with the maximum federal share of 80%. The purpose of the projects is to provide training and employment services to physically and mentally handicapped persons in a realistic work setting. Follow-up supportive services are often provided in conjunction with the project to assure handicapped individuals continuing employment opportunities in jobs for which they have been trained. Projects with Industry (PWI) was initially authorized under the 1968 amendments to the Vocational Rehabilitation Act.

The author was unable to identify any relevant MR/DD activities until FY 1978. Between FY 1978 and FY 1984, 17 MR/DD projects had been funded under Section 621. Grantees included public school systems, in-stitutions of higher education, private foundations, institutes, service organizations, workshops, and training centers. In FY 1982, 8 MR/DD projects out of a total of 15 projects were funded under Section 621. (See Table 34 for the funding history.)

PL 95-602, Section 316: Special Recreation Demonstrations

Section 316 authorizes grants to state agencies and to public or nonprofit organizations for the development of programs to provide handicapped individuals with recreational activities to aid in their mobility and socialization. Although the primary emphasis of this program is on services to physically handicapped individuals, mentally handicapped individuals also participate. About 15,000 people were served by FY 1982. The Reagan administration did not request funding in the president's budget for this program during FY 1981–84; however, Congress put money into it every year. In any given year approximately 200 applications are received but only an approximate total of 25 are funded. The number of total projects funded, with MR/DD projects listed in parentheses, are as follows: FY 1981, 25 projects (5); FY 1982, 23 projects (3); FY 1983, 27 projects (4); FY 1984, 27 projects (4). A total of 15 MR/DD projects have been funded since the program began in FY 1981. (See Table 34 for the funding history.)

BIOMEDICAL, BEHAVIORAL, AND HEALTH SERVICES RESEARCH

Public Health Services Act as Amended: NICHD and NINCDS

The profiles and sources of data for the research programs of the National Institute of Child Health and Human Development (NICHD) and the National Institute of Neurological and Communicative Disorders and Stroke (NINCDS) were described previously in this book. (See Chapter 4, Training of Biomedical and Health Services Personnel.) Trends in research funding at each institute are discussed next.

NICHD   In 1962, under PL 87-838, Title IV, Part E, Section 411 (the Public Health Services Act Amendments) the NICHD was established to investigate the biological, social, and behavioral bases of human development. Studies of physical, environmental, and psychological events that influence development are of primary concern. In 1983 budget hearings, the agency reported that it was funding 137 extramural research grants concerned with the epidemiology, etiology, diagnosis, prevention, and amelioration of mental retardation. These projects were being administered through the mental retardation branch of NICHD's Center for Research on Mothers and Children (CRMC). Representative contemporary extramural projects include studies of nutritional factors influencing prenatal development; research on prenatal diagnosis of PKU; an investigation on respiratory distress syndrome; and a study of the genetic basis of a specific learning disability. The study of prematurity and low birth weight infants is a ma-

jor focus of NICHD-funded research. The institute also conducts an active program of intramural research on mental retardation.

The NICHD funds the nation's largest program of research in mental retardation and developmental disabilities. NICHD presently supports 12 mental retardation research centers at the following sites across the country: Yeshiva University in New York, University of Washington in Seattle, University of Kansas at Lawrence, Universities of California at Los Angeles and San Francisco, Vanderbilt University (including George Peabody College, which was incorporated into Vanderbilt in 1980), University of North Carolina at Chapel Hill, University of Wisconsin at Madison, Children's Hospital Corporation in Boston, University of Colorado in Denver, Eunice K. Shriver Center for Mental Retardation, Inc. in Waltham, Massachusetts, and the University of Chicago. Funding for the Children's Hospital Research Foundation in Cincinnati was terminated in FY 1981 (J. Zagata, NICHD budget analyst, personal communication, January 14, 1985).

Annual funding for this research advanced consistently during FY 1964–79, climbing from $2.8 million to $29.2 million (see Figure 63). During FY 1979–84, MR/DD research funding was essentially flat. MR/DD research funding increased by an average of 1.4% per year over the entire 5-year span, but funding actually fell slightly in FY 1980–81—the first time this had occurred in the agency's 20-year history. A 12% increase in the agency's FY 1985 appropriation suggested that MR/DD research would also increase somewhat in FY 1985. Actual funding levels, however, are dependent on approved proposals selected for funding on a competitive basis.

Adjusting these figures to negate the impact of inflation revealed steady real growth during FY 1964–72, followed by a plateau in funding through FY 1979. MR/DD research funding then began the first period of general decline in the institute's history. Spending fell a total of 22% between FY 1979 and FY 1985 on an adjusted basis. The average rate of decline was 3.7% per year during this period.

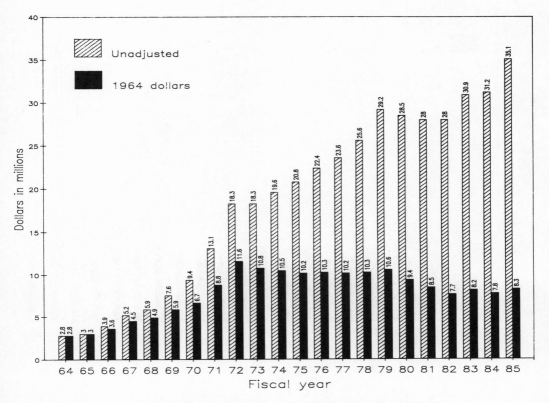

Figure 63. NICHD financial support for MR/DD research: FY 1964–85.

The recent decline in NICHD spending for MR/DD research has occurred in the context of slowed growth in the agency's total obligations. Total NICHD obligations have increased every year since FY 1964, except in FY 1973 and 1975 when the consistent growth was interrupted by the impounding (and later release) of funds. In the agency's first 8 years, between FY 1964 and FY 1972, the institute's budget almost quadrupled. Since then, growth of the NICHD's budget has slowed to an average of 9.4% per year. Adjusted for inflation, NICHD's budget increased steadily until peaking at $77.3 million in FY 1974. It remained at approximately that level through FY 1985 (see Figure 64).

The percentage of NICHD's budget devoted to MR/DD research has ranged from 7.1% in FY 1966 to a peak of 16.5% in FY 1975–76. Since then, there has been a constant decline. In FY 1985, only 11.2% of NICHD's budget

was devoted to MR/DD research. These trends are reflected in Figure 65. (See also Table 25 in Chapter 4.)

NINCDS The National Institute of Neurological, Communicative Disorders and Stroke was established under Title IV, Part D of the Public Health Services Act Amendments in 1950. The principal purposes of the institute include sponsoring fundamental neuroscientific research and studying the etiology, prevention, and cure of neurological problems and communicative disorders. Developmental disabilities often leading to mental retardation, such as cerebral palsy, epilepsy, spina bifida, and phenylketonuria, have been a major focus of NINCDS research since the creation of the institute. The institute funds a great deal of research on basic biological and molecular studies of the development and function of the nervous system.

The institute began supporting research re-

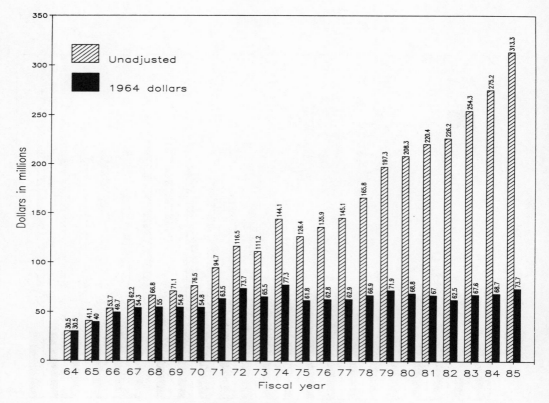

Figure 64.   NICHD budget history: FY 1964–85.

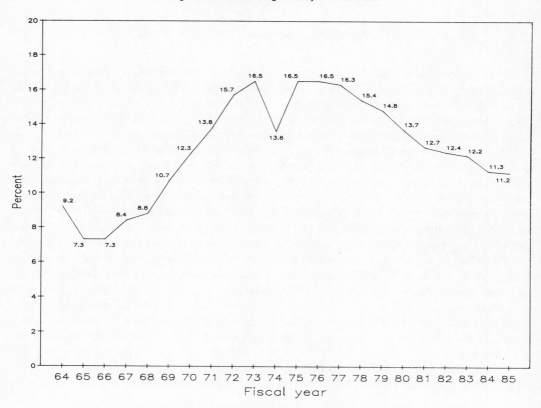

Figure 65.   Percentage of the NICHD total budget obligated for MR/DD research: FY 1964–85.

lated to MR/DD in FY 1954. One of the first studies it supported, along with NIMH and private foundations, was Masland, Sarason and Gladwin's comprehensive survey of research needs published in 1958 in *Mental Subnormality*. In 1958, the institute also initiated the first large-scale collaborative investigation of perinatal factors affecting mental and physical development in the United States. This study involved 50,000 mothers in 15 medical centers across the country. In FY 1983 House budget hearings, NINCDS was reported to be supporting 58 extramural investigations on MR/DD alone (U.S. House of Representatives [House], 1982).

In unadjusted terms, NINCDS support of MR/DD investigations rose every year between FY 1954 and FY 1968. Funding leveled off from FY 1968 to FY 1977 at about $5 million annually. Research spending increased by an average of 17.6% yearly during FY 1977–81 to $8.9 million; however, funding

regressed by FY 1985, to $7.67 million. This was a 4-year decline of 14% (see Figure 66).

Inflation had a considerable impact on these spending patterns. The adjusted figures registered major gains every year from FY 1954 to FY 1968, but declined by 48% during FY 1968–77, an average annual decrement of 5.5%. MR/DD spending climbed again during FY 1977–80, increasing by 12% per year. During FY 1980–85, however, research funding dropped at NINCDS by a total of 38% over the 6-year period. In real economic terms, in FY 1985, the institute was spending only slightly more per year on MR/DD research than it expended in FY 1960.

It should be noted that the decline in MR/DD expenditures was not occasioned by a decline in the overall spending of the institute (see Figure 67). MR/DD research spending was 5.3% of the institute's total obligations in FY 1972. In FY 1985, however, MR/DD research funding was projected to fall to 1.9%

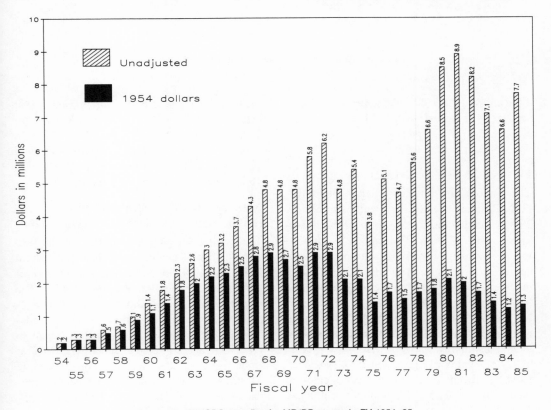

Figure 66. NINCDS spending for MR/DD research: FY 1954–85.

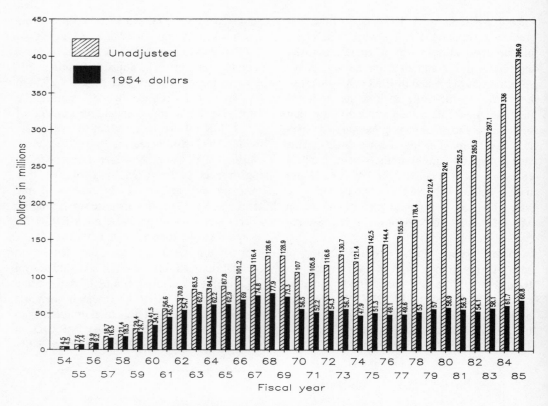

Figure 67.   NINCDS budget history (obligations): FY 1954–85.

of the enacted FY 1985 total appropriation for the agency, as illustrated in Figure 68. (See also Table 26 in Chapter 4.)

PL 81-962, Title IV: NIAID

The National Institute of Allergy and Infectious Diseases (NIAID) was authorized in the 1950 amendments to the Public Health Service Act (PL 81-962). The institute is supporting research in several areas intimately concerned with prevention of MR/DD and other disorders of the central nervous system in the fetus, newborn, and young child. Five areas of investigation funded by NIAID have great relevance to mental retardation and developmental disabilities: 1) Herpes Simplex Type 2; 2) Cytomegalovirus infections; 3) Toxoplasmosis; 4) Group "B" Streptococci, a cause of meningitis; and 5) Haemophilus Influenza Type "B," a cause of meningitis in children under 10 years of age.

On an unadjusted basis, funding advanced every year from $2.9 million in FY 1976, to $14.2 million in FY 1985 (see Table 35). On adjusted basis, funding growth averaged 12.4% annually between FY 1976 and FY 1985. These trends are depicted in Figure 69.

National Mental Health Act: NIMH (Public Health Services Act, Section 301)

The original legislative authority for the support of mental health research at the federal level is the National Mental Health Act of 1946, Title III, Section 301 (PL 79-487). The development of the National Institute of Mental Health research mission in mental retardation and developmental disabilities began in FY 1955; according to then NIMH Director Robert Felix, the agency was spending $146,000 on several projects in mental retardation research (Braddock, 1973). The following year, the FY 1956 HEW budget hearings before the House Subcommittee on

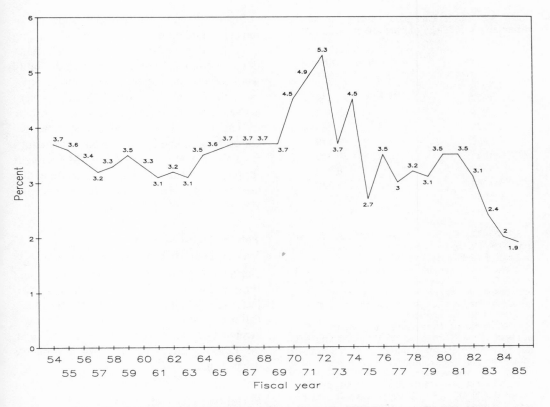

Figure 68. Percentage of the NINCDS total budget obligated for MR/DD research: FY 1954–85.

Labor-HEW Appropriations earmarked an increase of $250,000 over the FY 1955 NIMH appropriation and instructed the agency to spend it on mental retardation research (House, 1963, p. 2). The Senate sustained the recommendation and in FY 1956 NIMH actually obligated $923,000 on mental retardation projects.

For the next dozen years, FY 1955–67, NIMH was a major focal point for mental retardation research. Numerous NIMH research and research training projects were directly concerned with mental retardation and many others were indirectly relevant to it. Braddock (1973, p. 81), after an inspection of NIMH grant titles and project descriptions, indicated that mental retardation research during FY 1955–67 fell into three categories: 1) studies of learning, 2) analyses of the effects of cultural and social deprivation, and 3) studies of the behavioral and biological aspects of retardation.

Funding for NIMH research in mental retardation reached its zenith in FY 1963, the year the NICHD was created. The creation of the new institute brought about the transfer of NIMH basic research activity in child development. Four years later, in FY 1967, HEW was reorganized and certain key mental retardation activities were transferred to the newly created Social and Rehabilitation Service, Division on Mental Retardation. Beginning in FY 1969, NIMH MR/DD funding rapidly diminished. It fell to approximately $2 million annually for FY 1972–83 (see Table 36).

The record of hearings on the FY 1977 HEW budget indicates that "nine research projects are under way in the area of mental retardation and of this number four projects are being undertaken in the area of developmental studies" (OHI, 1976, February, p. 35). During FY 1979–83, however, only one project was identified by NIMH as having a "primary" focus on MR/DD. Funding for this project, the Phe-

Table 35. NIAID estimated funding for MR/DD research: FY 1976–85 (dollars are in thousands)

FY	MR/DD research funding
1976	$2,867
1977	$3,539
1978	$3,572
1979	$3,860
1980	$6,119
1981	$6,340
1982	$6,849
1983	$10,810
1984	$12,192
1985	$14,166

Source: The FY 1980 House appropriations hearings (U.S. House of Representatives [House], 1979, p. 593) presented data on NIAID expenditures and discussed the institute's research program relevant to MR/DD. This, however, is the only published or unpublished reference to NIAID-sponsored MR/DD research identified during the course of the author's analysis of federal spending.

Dr. John Nutter, NIAID, chief of programming and evaluation, was contacted for further information (personal communication, January 16, 1984). It was concluded that the five infectious agents aforementioned in this section were the focus of the agency's research most relevant to MR/DD. NIAID staff confirmed the NIAID MR/DD expenditure figures presented in the record of the FY 1980 House appropriation hearings (House, 1979) and provided additional data for FY 1979–84. FY 1985 data were also provided by Nutter (personal communication, November, 1984); he also stated that he was certain that NIAID was sponsoring research related to the five infectious agents prior to FY 1976, but no figures could be provided without a search of agency files. The agency declined to do this due to inadequate manpower.

nylketonuria Collaborative Study, was terminated in FY 1983.

In real economic terms, NIMH mental retardation support rose almost continuously on an annual basis from FY 1955 to FY 1963. Support for mental retardation then generally declined, falling in 2 years to only half the FY 1963 level. Funding plateaued on an adjusted basis around the $2 million level through the rest of the 1960s. In the 1970s, adjusted funding levels showed a dramatic decline of 71%, falling to $.68 million in FY 1979. By FY 1983, support for mental retardation projects in real economic terms was less than 10% of the FY 1963 peak.

Figure 70 reflects financial support for mental retardation projects only. Including projects in accord with the PL 95-602 functional definition of developmental disability would require the author's analysis to incorporate other research in which NIMH is very active—such as research on severe chronic mental illness in which onset may have occurred prior to age 22. House budget hearings for FY 1985 also referred to NIMH support for projects related to autism and learning disorders (U.S. House of Representatives, 1984).

Public Health Services Act, Section 303: HIP and HIST

During FY 1964–67, Hospital Improvement Projects and Hospital In-service Training Projects were administered by the NIMH. After that period, they were transferred to the newly created Social and Rehabilitation Service in the DHEW. (See Chapter 4 for a complete discussion.)

Social Security Act, Title V, Section 512: Health Services Research

Health services research is indirectly tied to the nation's first health services formula grant program, enacted in 1921, which was the predecessor of today's Maternal and Child Health (MCH) and Crippled Children's (CC) Services Programs. The original act operated until 1928, and was known as the Sheppard-Towner Act, or the Maternity and Infancy Act. In 1935, this legislation was expanded under Title V of the Social Security Act (PL 74-271). This legislation initiated the Crippled Children's Services Program and established a special fund for demonstration projects in the training of personnel.

In 1963, acting on several of the recommendations of President Kennedy's Panel on Mental Retardation, Congress enacted PL 88-156, the Maternal and Child Health and Mental Retardation Planning Act of 1963. This law formally established the research program under Section 512 to support studies "which show promise of substantial contribu-

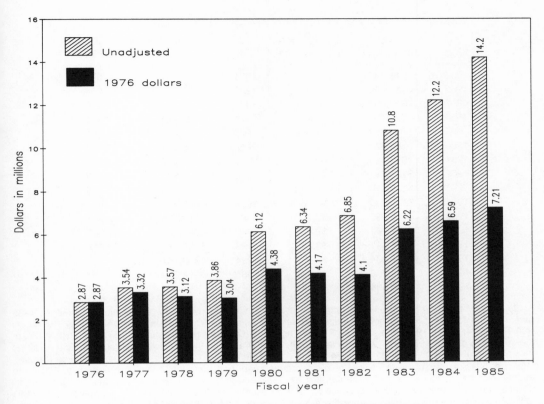

Figure 69.   NIAID research spending relevant to MR/DD: FY 1976–85.

tion to the advancement'' of MCH/CC Services (Braddock, 1973, p. 85).

The Social Security Amendments of 1967 (PL 90-248) consolidated MCH/CC Services funding under a single grant authorization, with a funding split of 50% for formula grants, 40% for project grants, and 10% for national research and training projects. On July 1, 1974, PL 92-345 stipulated that funding for project grants in the states was to be added to the state formula grant allocations. This meant that 90% of the program's total appropriation would be allocated directly to the states through the formula grant program. States were, however, required to include in their state plans provisions for conducting activities similar to those previously authorized under the special fund for demonstration projects. (The 10% component allocated for national research and training projects continued to be awarded by the department through project grants.)

Effective October 1, 1982, the Maternal and Child Health Services Block Grant Program became law, consolidating the MCH/CC formula grant program with several other categorical health services grant programs. Fifteen percent of the block grant must be set aside for all special projects including research and training.

Figure 71 depicts the funding history for MR/DD projects under Section 512 of the MCH/CC Services research authority. Funding peaked in FY 1968–69 at $2 million in unadjusted terms (see Table 37). Then, funds plateaued at $1.6 million during FY 1971–74 and then again during FY 1975–80 at $1.28 million. After the Omnibus Budget Reconciliation Act's implementation, MR/DD research spending plummeted even more severely than in previous years. Obligations for mental retardation and developmental disabilities dropped by 77% in FY 1981, to a 20-year low of $300,000. MR/DD research funding con-

Table 36.　NIMH funding: FY 1955–85 (dollars are in thousands)

FY	Total expenditures	Sec. 301 MR expenditures	FY	Total expenditures	Sec. 301 MR expenditures
1955	$11,759	$146	1971	$342,542	$3,505
1956	$17,958	$923	1972	$377,084	$2,034
1957	$30,006	$1,630	1973	$379,285	$1,475
1958	$38,457	$1,947	1974	$387,921	$751
1959	$49,853	$2,356	1975	$418,023	$1,966
1960	$67,470	$2,808	1976[a]	$486,571	$2,157
1961	$91,923	$3,947	1977	$450,527	$2,014
1962	$107,711	$5,275	1978	$500,341	$2,173
1963	$139,517	$5,743	1979	$569,835	$2,476
1964	$170,990	$3,280	1980	$562,809	$2,032
1965	$186,067	$2,730	1981	$532,366	$2,208
1966	$259,241	$2,905	1982	$229,049	$1,943
1967	$304,341	$3,211	1983	$225,985	$2,098
1968	$327,204	$4,300	1984	$253,157	
1969	$306,798	$4,888	1985	$279,002	
1970	$296,684	$4,295			

Source: FY 1955–72 data are from Braddock (1973, p. 80). Mental retardation expenditures for FY 1973–83 are from the following House appropriations hearings materials: FY 1973 data are from FY 1975 hearings (OMRC, 1974, p. 61); 1974 data are from FY 1976 hearings (Office for Handicapped Individuals [OHI], 1975, p. 66); FY 1975 data are from FY 1977 hearings (OHI, 1976, p. 8); FY 1976–78 data are from FY 1980 hearings (House, 1979, p. 591); 1980–83 data are from FY 1983 hearings (U.S. House of Representatives [House], 1983, p. 521). According to the NIMH financial management unit (personal communication, July, 1983), no mental retardation funds were identifiable after FY 1983 and indeed none appeared in the FY 1984 DHHS House budget hearings materials (U.S. House of Representatives [House], 1983). To paraphrase an NIMH official: Mental retardation activities are the responsibility of the NICHD and HDS (the Human Development Services Office in DHHS).

The mental retardation estimates in the table include funding for research and training activities because it was possible only during FY 1972–75 to separate these funds from one another. The large majority of these funds, however, supported research activities. Data for FY 1973–75 indicated that two-thirds of the mental retardation funds were expended for research, one-third for training. See also House hearings (House, 1963, pp. 1–4) for documentation that funds were spent primarily for research prior to FY 1963.

All mental retardation figures in the table exclude Hospital Improvement Project (HIP) and Hospital In-Service Training (HIST) Project funding under Section 303 of the Public Health Service Act.

Total NIMH obligations for FY 1955–65 are from Braddock (1973, p. 80). Data for FY 1966–85 were provided by the NIMH Budget Office (D. Gurwitz, personal communication, February 13, 1985).

[a]Includes transition quarter.

tinued to decline in FY 1982–83, falling to $200,000 and $150,000, respectively. In FY 1984 and FY 1985, MR/DD spending was pegged at $290,000. In adjusted dollars, funding declined every year during FY 1968–83.

Total unadjusted appropriations for all Section 512 research activities peaked in FY 1969–70 at $6.2 million, plateaued at $6 million in FY 1972–74, then remained constant at $5.4 million during FY 1975–80. Figure 72 displays trends in overall funding for Section

512 research. In real economic terms, Section 512 funding in FY 1984 was 33% below the FY 1980 level and slightly below the initial level of funding in FY 1964. The percentage of total Section 512 research obligations constituted by MR/DD studies ranged between 37% (in FY 1967) and 24% (in FY 1980) during FY 1965–80. Since the implementation of the Block Grant in FY 1982, that percentage has declined precipitously to between 7.7% and 3.9% (see Figure 73).

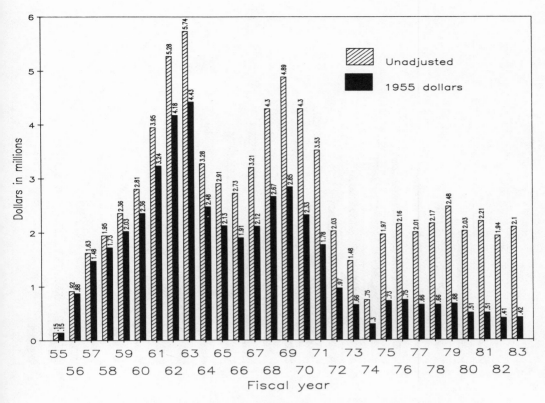

Figure 70.   Mental retardation research funded by NIMH, under Section 301: FY 1955–83.

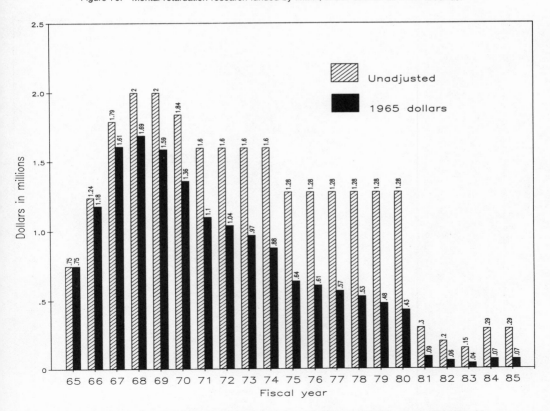

Figure 71.   Maternal and Child Health Services research funding for MR/DD projects: FY 1965–85.

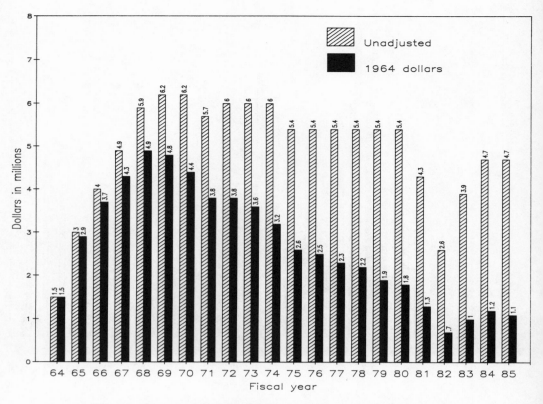

Figure 72.   Maternal and Child Health Services total research funding: FY 1964–85.

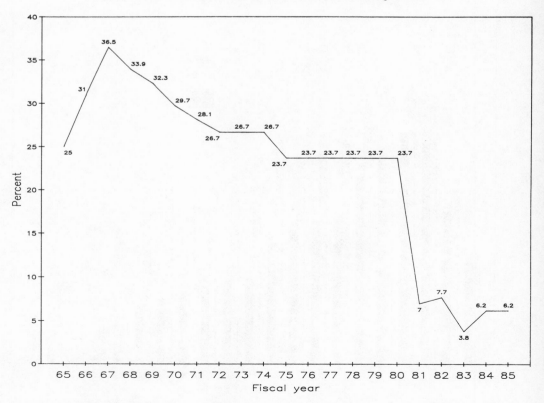

Figure 73.   MR/DD research funding as a percentage of total Maternal and Child Health Services research funding under Section 512 and the Block Grant: FY 1965–85.

Table 37.   Section 512 research funding: FY 1964–
85 (dollars are in thousands)

FY	MR/DD research	Total research
1964		$1,500
1965	$750	$3,000
1966	$1,240	$4,000
1967	$1,791	$4,900
1968	$2,000	$5,900
1969	$2,000	$6,200
1970	$1,842	$6,200
1971	$1,600	$5,735
1972	$1,600	$6,035
1973	$1,600	$6,035
1974	$1,600	$6,035
1975	$1,280	$5,354
1976	$1,280	$5,354
1977	$1,280	$5,354
1978	$1,280	$5,354
1979	$1,280	$5,354
1980	$1,280	$5,354
1981	$300	$4,300
1982	$200	$2,600
1983	$150	$3,900
1984	$290	$4,700
1985	$290	$4,700

Source: FY 1964–72 data are from Braddock (1973, p. 83). FY 1973–74 data are from FY 1975 House hearings (OMRC, 1974, p. 61). FY 1975–76 data are from FY 1976 House hearings (OHI, 1975, p. 66). No breakout was available on MR/DD research support levels after FY 1976.

Because MR/DD has historically had 25%–33% of total Section 512 funds devoted to it, MCH agency officials believe that funds were still being deployed for MR/DD research projects at a relatively similar priority level from 1977 to 1980 (R. Hornmuth, personal communication, November 29, 1983). In addition, the FY 1976 House budget hearings (OHI, 1975) reported that $1.28 million would be expended for MR/DD research that year. Data for FY 1981–84 were provided by Dr. Gontran Lamberty, director, MCH research program (personal communication, December 7, 1984). Projections for FY 1985 were not available. The author's figure assumes continuation at the same level as FY 1984. Jim Papai, MCH, Office of Research and Training (personal communication, December 7, 1984) said that was a reasonable assumption given the fact that total Section 512 appropriations for FY 1985 remained at the FY 1984 level.

Chapter 6

Income Maintenance Programs

FEDERAL INCOME MAINTENANCE programs for disabled persons in the United States stem from four major legislative achievements: 1) enactment of the original Social Security Act of 1935, with its provisions for aged persons, dependent children, and blind persons contained in Titles I, IV, and X, respectively; 2) authorization in 1950 of the Title XIV Aid to the Permanently and Totally Disabled Program (APTD); 3) passage of the Social Security Amendments of 1956, authorizing benefits for Adult Disabled Children (ADC) through the Old Age, Survivors, and Disability Insurance (OASDI) Trust Fund; and 4) establishment, via the Social Security Amendments of 1972, of the Supplemental Security Income (SSI) Program under Title XVI, which extended benefits to children and federalized administration of the program. Congress passed Food Stamp Act Amendments in 1979 to authorize stamps for residents of community living facilities. The composition of FY 1985 federal income maintenance for persons with mental retardation is depicted in Figure 74.

Federal income maintenance spending was the principal fiscal component of the federal mission in mental retardation for the 27-year period of FY 1950–76. Funds allocated for this purpose rose from $2.5 million to $1.1 billion during the period. Prior to FY 1950, there were no federal expenditures for income maintenance payments solely on the basis of mental retardation. Spending for mental retardation services first surpassed the volume of funds budgeted for income maintenance payments to this population in FY 1973 and has

done so continuously since FY 1977. In FY 1985, projected total income maintenance payments were $3 billion, nearly tripling in unadjusted terms over the past 8 years. An additional $444,000 and $978,000 in FY 1985 were projected to be expended from SSI and OASDI trust funds, respectively, for rehabilitation services authorized under Title XVI, Section 1615 and Title II, Section 222 of the Social Security Act.

In real economic terms, total federal income maintenance spending for individuals with mental retardation grew 34% in the 1950s, 12% in the 1960s, and 10% in the 1970s. From FY 1980 to FY 1985, the real growth rate slowed to an average annual rate of 2.2%, and declined by 1.9% in FY 1982. The historical growth of federal income maintenance spending to persons with mental retardation from FY 1950 to FY 1985 is illustrated in Figures 75–77.

APPROPRIATED FUNDS

Social Security Act, Title XIV: Aid to the Permanently and Totally Disabled

The Aid to the Permanently and Totally Disabled Program, commonly known as APTD, was authorized in 1950. Before APTD's adoption, nonaged disabled persons, excluding blind persons, were ineligible for federal public assistance. To receive public assistance, individuals with mental retardation had to receive "General Assistance," which was not federally aided, but was financed by state and local administrative units. In most states, the

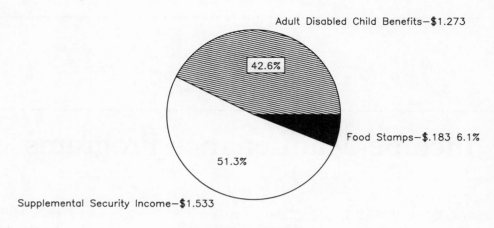

Total: $2.990 Billion

Figure 74.   Federal income maintenance spending for persons with mental retardation: FY 1985. (Dollars are in billions.)

legal basis for General Assistance was derived from the Elizabethan Poor Laws, and was sufficiently broad to include any needy person except nonresidents.

General Assistance   According to the Calhoun Report (U.S. House of Representatives [House], 1946), General Assistance Programs in FY 1945 were administered throughout the

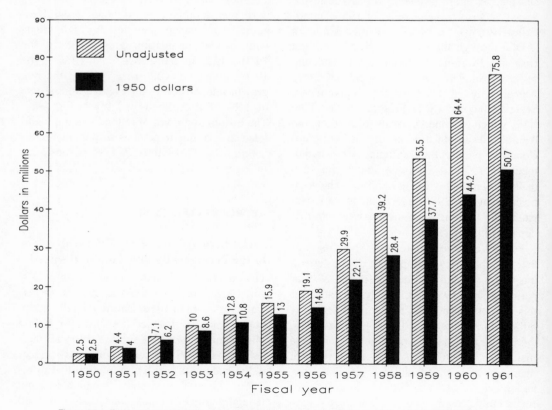

Figure 75.   Federal income maintenance expenditures for persons with mental retardation: FY 1950–61.

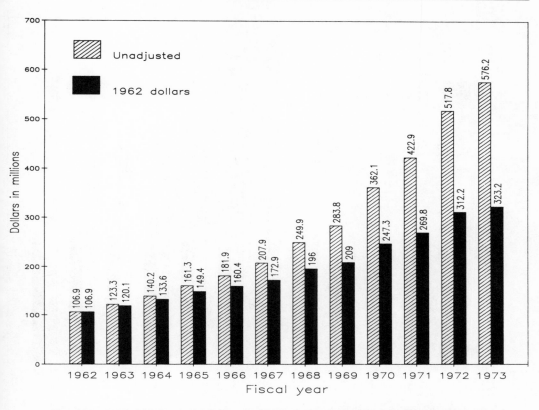

Figure 76. Federal income maintenance expenditures for persons with mental retardation: FY 1962–73.

United States by more than 10,000 local administrative units (e.g., counties, villages, and towns). Eligibility and amount of assistance varied with each independent administrative unit. In states with limited fiscal strength, the opportunity to receive matching federal funds (for "the Blind," "the Aged," or for "Dependent Children" only) restricted rather than increased the availability of state and local funds for General Assistance. So long as General Assistance Programs remained outside the scope of federal grants-in-aid, they were at a considerable financial disadvantage. In FY 1944, in a survey of 44 states, 14 states assumed no financial responsibility at all for General Assistance and 3 others contributed less than 3% of the cost; in 27 states, the state carried half the cost of General Assistance (House, 1946). Local funds met only 7% of the total cost of Old-Age Assistance in the United States in FY 1944,

about 10% of the cost of Aid to the Blind, and about 18% of the cost of Aid to Dependent Children. For General Assistance, however, the local share was 52%.

The average payment for General Assistance in June, 1945, according to the Calhoun Report, was $29 per case, per month. Payment averages per case ranged from $45 in New York to $9 in Mississippi. In the summer of 1945, 19 large cities with 20% of the United States population had 33% of the General Assistance cases in the entire country. These 19 cities paid 45% of the total funds expended that year for the amount of General Assistance. The Calhoun Report noted that, "General Assistance is extremely meager in some counties and in others totally lacking" (House, 1946, p. 301). The 19 cities were: Baltimore, Boston, Buffalo, Chicago, Cincinnati, Cleveland, Detroit, Washington, D.C., Los Angeles, Milwaukee, Minneapolis, New-

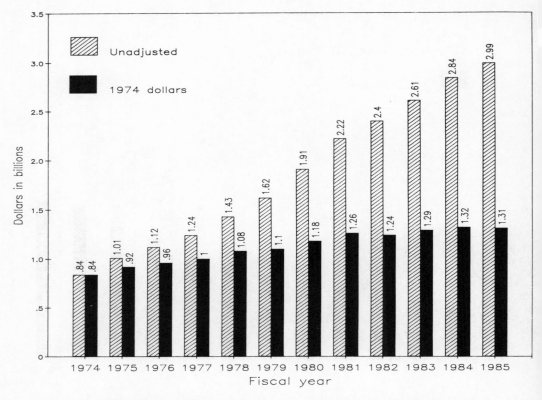

Figure 77. Federal income maintenance expenditures for persons with mental retardation: FY 1974–85.

ark, New Orleans, New York, Philadelphia, Pittsburgh, Rochester, St. Louis, and San Francisco.

APTD The public assistance component of the original Social Security Act of 1935 contained no provisions for assisting disabled individuals, other than a small program for Aid to the Blind, which was authorized in Title X. In addition to Aid to the Blind, Old-Age Assistance (Title I) and Aid to Families with Dependent Children (Title IV) were also established in the original act. A decade after the implementation of the act, the staff of the House Committee on Ways and Means described the major limitations of the original Social Security legislation as follows:

> In addition to the inadequacies due to established maximums and fiscal inequalities among states, the Social Security Act completely fails to provide for some need. Needy persons for whom there is no federal provision include: 1) dependent children not qualified under present defini-

tions for Aid to Dependent Children; 2) persons excluded from assistance because of residence provisions; 3) the catch-all group defined as "general assistance" recipients which include (a) childless widows under 65 years, (b) infirm, ill, or disabled persons other than blind, under 65 years, and (c) employable persons who cannot find work. (House, 1946, p. 312)

In 1950, Congress responded to these deficiencies by enacting amendments to the Social Security Act that established the APTD Program under Title XIV. Broad latitude was given to the states in terms of standards required for program eligibility. However, federal regulations specified that each state's public assistance plan must contain a definition of permanently and totally disabled in which "permanently" was related to the degree of disability. Over the next 25 years, minor changes in the APTD Program were implemented but the state-run, federally assisted character of the program remained in-

Table 38. APTD payments to persons with mental retardation: FY 1950–73 (dollars are in thousands)

FY	Total payments June	Total payments × 12 months	Total recipients	MR payments	MR % primary & secondary diagnosis	MR recipients
1950	$2,655	$31,860	62,666	$2,485	7.8%	4,887
1951	$4,677	$56,124	104,000	$4,377	7.8%	8,112
1952	$6,695	$80,340	145,000	$7,069	8.8%	12,760
1953	$8,498	$101,976	176,000	$9,993	9.8%	17,248
1954	$9,931	$119,172	209,000	$12,870	10.8%	22,572
1955	$11,260	$135,120	234,000	$15,944	11.8%	27,612
1956	$12,465	$149,580	255,000	$19,146	12.8%	32,640
1957	$14,399	$172,788	281,000	$23,844	13.8%	38,778
1958	$16,393	$196,716	311,000	$29,113	14.8%	46,028
1959	$18,129	$217,548	336,000	$34,372	15.8%	53,088
1960	$19,617	$235,404	358,000	$39,547	16.8%	60,144
1961	$21,250	$255,000	378,000	$45,390	17.8%	67,284
1962	$23,530	$282,360	409,000	$50,824	18.0%	73,620
1963	$26,370	$316,440	448,000	$57,908	18.3%	81,984
1964	$29,668	$356,016	484,000	$65,506	18.4%	89,056
1965	$34,691	$416,292	536,000	$77,430	18.6%	99,696
1966	$39,996	$479,952	573,000	$90,230	18.8%	107,724
1967	$47,254	$567,048	615,000	$106,605	18.8%	116,850
1968	$54,301	$651,612	670,000	$125,109	19.2%	128,640
1969	$64,692	$776,304	755,000	$149,826	19.3%	145,715
1970	$83,885	$1,006,620	878,000	$194,161	19.3%	169,454
1971	$97,442	$1,169,304	995,000	$225,675	19.3%	192,035
1972	$113,410	$1,360,920	1,136,000	$262,657	19.3%	219,248
1973	$130,653	$1,567,836	1,211,000	$302,592	19.3%	233,723

Source: Estimates of the participation of persons with mental retardation in the APTD Program are based on three studies. The first one is the 1951 APTD characteristics study, which noted that 6.5% of all APTD recipients had "mental deficiency" (U.S. Department of Health, Education, and Welfare [DHEW], 1955, May, p. 13). The second study was conducted in November, 1964, and published in the *Welfare in Review* (Mugge, 1964). Mugge identified the MR participation rate as 14.7% in 1962. Litvin and Browning (1977) cited this study and indicated that it referred to persons with a primary diagnosis of mental retardation on APTD rolls. An added 3% of recipients had a secondary diagnosis of mental retardation. Finally, Braddock (1973) cited a 1970 Adult Characteristics Study of the APTD recipients, which indicated that persons with a primary or secondary diagnosis of mental retardation amounted to 16% and 3.3%, respectively, of the total APTD population for a total MR rate of 19.3%.

Based on discussions with the DHHS Social Security Administration, Office of Family Assistance (E. Dye, personal communications, February, 1985) recipient rate estimates were adjusted to reflect gradual increases in the rate over the 23-year period, using the fixed data points for 1951, 1962, and 1970 as benchmarks. All mental retardation payment levels, including those for 1950–61, include recipients with a primary or secondary diagnosis of mental retardation. A secondary diagnosis of mental retardation constituted 20% of primary diagnoses in the 1962 and 1970 characteristics studies. Thus, the 1951 primary and secondary rate was estimated to be 12.0% of the ascertained 1951 recipients with a primary diagnosis (6.5% × 1.2 = 7.8%). (Note: APTD recipient statistics were collected on a monthly basis. This table employs these monthly recipient statistics to impute levels of mental retardation spending on a fiscal year basis.)

tact. The number of individuals with a primary or secondary diagnosis of mental retardation receiving assistance grew from an estimated 27,612 in FY 1955 to 233,723 in FY 1973 (see Table 38). In FY 1974, the program was superseded by the SSI Program, which had been authorized by the 1972 amendments to the Social Security Act.

Figure 78 displays the steady increase in estimated APTD payments to persons with mental retardation, culminating in a payment level of $302.6 million in FY 1973. Payments

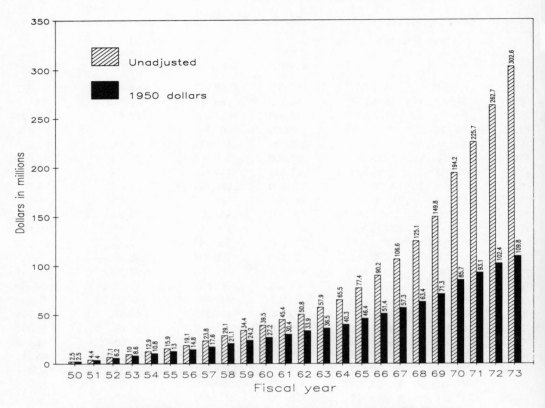

Figure 78.   APTD Program payments to persons with mental retardation: FY 1950–73.

to persons with mental retardation grew at an average annual rate of 19% for the 10-year period of FY 1964–73. The comparable growth rate for the entire APTD Program was 18%; the impact of inflation reduced these rates by about 50%.

Social Security Act, Title XVI: Supplemental Security Income

The Social Security Amendments of 1972 (PL 92-603) repealed the existing public assistance programs for elderly, blind, and disabled persons and added a new Title XVI to the act. Title XVI authorized a consolidated, federally administered program of cash benefits for needy adults. Under the SSI Program, a basic federal income support level was established for aged, blind, and disabled persons. Eligibility was to be determined and benefits paid by the federal government, acting through the

Social Security Administration. States were permitted to supplement the basic federal income support levels on behalf of selected classes of recipients, and in FY 1984, 45 states and the District of Columbia did so.

It is important to distinguish between the SSI Program and the Adult Disabled Child (ADC) Program under Social Security. SSI cash payments are available only to aged, blind, and disabled persons who meet a statutory test of financial need. SSI payments derive from general appropriations. ADC benefits, authorized under Title II, Section 202(d), are derived from a special OASDI trust fund financed through Social Security taxes paid by covered workers and their employers. The definition of disability adopted for the SSI Program follows the definition in Title II of the Social Security Act, which authorizes the ADC Program. Disability must begin prior to age 22 and meet a statutory test of severity that precludes "substantial gainful activity" (SGA).

Under SSI, disabled and blind children under 18 years of age were, for the first time, eligible for benefits, provided that their disabilities were of comparable severity to adult recipients. Under SSI's provisions, however, an eligible individual who is living in a state-operated institution or in a public or private health care facility which receives substantial payments on his or her behalf under Medicaid has his or her federal benefits reduced to a personal needs allowance of $25 per month. If an eligible individual is living in "the household of another" and receives support and maintenance from that person, the SSI basic payment amount is reduced by one-third.

Federal SSI payments to persons with mental retardation on an unadjusted basis advanced from $512 million in FY 1974 to a projected $1.532 billion in FY 1985 (see Table 39). Growth was particularly rapid in the 1970s, averaging 12% per year. However, the rate of growth slowed appreciably during the 1980s, falling to an average annual rate of 8% between FY 1981 and FY 1985.

In real economic terms, the fiscal trends are quite different (see Figure 79). The average annual rate of growth during FY 1974–80 was only 3.2%. The FY 1981–85 period was essentially flat, exhibiting a growth rate of 1.8%. Payment levels actually fell, but by less than a percentage point in FY 1978 and FY 1982. The FY 1985 figure was 3% below the FY 1984 payment level, but it is based on projections that may not accurately predict actual FY 1985 spending levels.

Payment Levels Monthly payment rates to individuals and to couples are adjusted annually to account for changes in the cost of living. In FY 1984, eligible disabled individuals averaged $257 per month, ranging from $201 in South Dakota to $285 in New York. In calculating an individual's eligibility, the Social Security Administration "disregards" the initial $20 of monthly income an individual receives from any source and up to $65 of any additional "earned" income. Any additional unearned income an applicant or re-

cipient receives each month results in a dollar-for-dollar reduction in his or her SSI benefit. "Earned" income above the original disregard ($65 a month; or up to $85, if the individual has no unearned income) causes a $1 reduction in the benefit payment for every $2 of additional earnings. In addition to meeting this income test, an individual cannot have personal resources that exceed certain statutory limits, such as a savings account exceeding $1,500 or an expensive home. This asset limit is being gradually raised to $2,000 by FY 1989.

The SSI program is legislatively linked with the Vocational Rehabilitation Program under Section 1615 of the Social Security Act. Adults under 65 years of age who are receiving SSI must be referred to the state vocational rehabilitation agency. Childhood recipients under age 16 must be referred to the designated state SSI disabled children's agency, usually the Crippled Children's Agency. Adult SSI recipients may not without good cause refuse rehabilitation services. The services provided to SSI recipients through state vocational rehabilitation agencies are reimbursed by the federal government out of special funds set aside for this purpose. PL 97-35 (Omnibus Budget Reconciliation Act), enacted August 13, 1981, stipulated that disabled beneficiaries had to engage in substantial gainful activity for 9 continuous months for federal reimbursements to be provided.

Amendments to the Social Security Act also included PL 94-566, which contained the "Keys Amendment," eliminating a major disincentive in the development of community facilities for persons with mental retardation by excluding publicly operated community residences serving 16 or fewer individuals from the definition of a public institution. Section 505 of these amendments also stipulated that assistance furnished on the basis of need to an SSI applicant by a state or local government would not be counted as unearned income for purposes of determining SSI eligibility or payment level. Under the previous law only certain types of public payments were disregarded, such as SSI "state supplemental

Table 39. SSI recipients and payments: FY 1974–85 (dollars are in thousands)

FY	Total federal payments	Federal payments to blind and disabled	Estimated MR SSI federal payments	Total recipients of federal payments	Blind and disabled recipients of federal payments	Estimated MR recipients of federal payments	Blind and disabled recipients of federal or federal & state payments	Estimated MR recipients of federal or federal & state payments
1974	$3,833,161	$2,050,420	$512,606	2,955,959	1,265,463	316,366	1,719,850	429,963
1975	$4,313,538	$2,470,558	$617,639	3,893,419	1,868,654	467,164	2,025,940	506,485
1976	$4,512,061	$2,727,065	$681,766	3,799,069	1,931,751	482,938	2,110,192	527,523
1977	$4,703,292	$2,966,480	$741,620	3,777,856	2,012,709	503,177	2,009,354	552,388
1978	$4,880,691	$3,174,471	$793,617	3,754,663	2,069,012	517,253	2,289,173	567,293
1979	$5,279,181	$3,519,753	$879,938	3,687,119	2,093,633	523,408	2,298,935	574,733
1980	$5,866,354	$4,006,161	$1,001,540	3,682,411	2,149,045	537,261	2,355,269	588,817
1981	$6,517,727	$4,550,702	$1,137,678	3,590,103	2,160,232	540,058	2,359,723	589,930
1982	$6,907,043	$4,902,313	$1,225,578	3,473,301	2,143,816	535,094	2,328,942	582,235
1983	$7,422,524	$5,388,098	$1,347,024	3,589,521	2,250,428	562,607	2,409,042	602,260
1984	$8,142,171	$5,964,498	$1,491,125	3,698,758	2,352,047	588,011	2,521,991	630,498
1985	$8,399,000	$6,131,270	$1,532,828					

Source: To determine the estimated number of recipients with mental retardation of SSI, staff at the Social Security Administration (SSA) Office of Research, Statistics and International Policy were consulted. The procedure ultimately adopted is based on the results of an unpublished SSA study. The 1981 study matched newly awarded recipients in FY 1977 to those still receiving payments 4 years later. By matching these two data sets, the diagnosis of present recipients can be determined. Routinely, diagnostic information is collected only at the time of application and is not carried in the computerized "master record" payment files.

The 1981 study indicated that 25% of all blind and disabled SSI recipients were diagnosed as mentally retarded. SSI payments to persons with mental retardation were then estimated on the basis of this prevalence statistic applied to the total payments to blind and disabled SSI recipients (J. Schmulowitz, SSA, director of the Division of Statistics and Analysis, Statistics and International Policy, Office of Research, personal communications, June, 1983). Payment data for FY 1974–83 for blind and disabled recipients were obtained from the "Social Security Bulletin, Annual Statistical Supplement" (U.S. Department of Health and Human Services [DHHS], 1983). Data for FY 1984 were provided by Richard Bell, (personal communication, November 26, 1984). The FY 1985 data are the budget authority figures approved by Congress as provided by Aaron Stopak and Neil Nieman, SSA, Office of Management, Budget, and Personnel (personal communication, November 15, 1984).

Recipient counts include those persons receiving only federal SSI payments plus those receiving federal SSI in combination with a federally administered or state administered state supplement. Persons who receive only a state supplement are not included in the table. The FY 1974–83 data were obtained from Table 161 of the "Social Security Bulletin, Annual Statistical Supplement" (DHHS, 1983). The FY 1984 data were provided by Bell (personal communication, Feburary 25, 1985). The FY 1985 data were provided by the SSA Office of Management and Budget (personal communication, November 15, 1984). They represent budget authority figures for FY 1985 approved by Congress.

The inclusion of children under 18 years of age in the SSI Program in FY 1974, coupled with an elevation in payment levels, had an immediate impact on public assistance funds expended for persons with mental retardation that year. FY 1974 obligations to this group under the new and expanded SSI Program were slightly in excess of $500 million, an unadjusted gain of 70% over the previous year's level. Some of this increase may be attributed to the analytic techniques used to compute mental retardation expenditures during the APTD/SSI transition. A great deal of the increase, however, was due to the

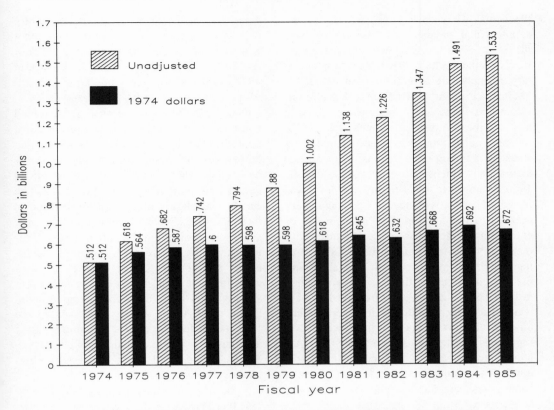

Figure 79.   Estimated federal SSI payments to persons with mental retardation: FY 1974–85.

payments'' and payments for medical care and social services.

PL 94-566 also repealed the controversial Section 1616(E) of the Social Security Act which called for a dollar-for-dollar reduction in the federal SSI payment to an individual when a state made a supplemental payment on behalf of any eligible resident in a facility providing services that could have been financed under the state's Medicaid program. The 1976 amendments substituted a new provision requiring states to establish and enforce standards governing care in nonmedical facilities housing a ''significant number'' of SSI recipients. The Social Security Disability Amendments of 1980, PL 96-265, extended the trial work period during which SSI benefits may not be terminated for 24 months, and authorized work incentive and other demonstration projects. On October 9, 1984, President Reagan signed into law the Social Se-

curity Disability Benefits Reform Act. The act reauthorized through June 30, 1978, a provision of existing law, Section 1619 (a) and (b), permitting certain severely disabled SSI recipients to continue receiving special federal income maintenance payments and Medicaid-financed health care services even though their earnings exceed the applicable test of substantial gainful activity.

Procedures to inhibit the arbitrary removal of beneficiaries from the SSI and SSDI Programs' rolls were also strengthened in the Social Security Disability Benefits Reform Act of 1984. The act stipulated that the DHHS Secretary can only authorize termination of benefits if there is evidence of medical improvement in the individual's impairment and the individual is able to engage in substantial gainful activity.

State Supplementary Payments States have the option of supplementing federal SSI payments. They may either administer the supplemental payments themselves or have the Social Security Administration make payments on their behalf. When state supplementary payments are federally administered, the Social Security Administration makes eligibility and payment determinations for the state and assumes administrative costs. In 1976, federal legislation was enacted, requiring states to maintain their optional state supplementation payments at the level of December, 1976, when the federal SSI payment level was increased. Effective June, 1982, states were allowed to switch from the "maintenance of expenditures method" of compliance with mandatory pass through (described above) to the "payment level" method, by maintaining the rates in effect for the December previous to the change. In 1983, the pass through law was adjusted by substituting state supplementary payment levels in effect in March, 1983, for those in effect in December, 1976. Although laws have prevented states from reducing their supplements, unlike federal SSI payments, state supplements generally have not kept pace with the rate of inflation.

In FY 1984, 23 states and the District of Columbia had federally administered state supplementary payments, 22 states had state administered state supplements, and 5 states (Maryland, New Mexico, Texas, Utah, and West Virginia) did not supplement federal SSI payments.

PL 95-113: Food Stamp Aid

The first federal Food Stamp Program was established as an experiment in 1939, for the dual purpose of stabilizing food prices by removing surplus agricultural commodities from the market and feeding poor families. The program concluded with World War II, but was revived in 1961, again as an experimental project, in a few areas of the country. The pilot project was expanded during the "War on Poverty" and enacted into law as the Food Stamp Act of 1964. Amendments to the act in 1971 established uniform federal eligibility standards and coupon values. In 1973, Con-

gress mandated that all areas of the country offer food stamps and convert from other federal food distribution programs. A major revision of the Food Stamp Act took place in 1977, with the enactment of PL 95-113. PL 95-113 was particularly significant for individuals with MR/DD because it permitted public assistance offices to determine client eligibility for food stamps. This meant that households composed entirely of SSI recipients could apply for food stamps at Social Security Administration branch offices and be certified as eligible, based on information in their SSI files. The act also required the state agency administering the Food Stamp Program to notify SSI recipients about the availability and benefits of the Food Stamp Program, as well as eligibility requirements.

Two years later, the Food Stamp Amendments of 1970 for the first time authorized food stamps for residents of community living arrangements for blind and disabled persons. The amendments, PL 96-58, redefined "eligible households" to include:

> Disabled or blind recipients of benefits under Title II or Title XVI of the Social Security Act who are residents in a public or private nonprofit group living arrangement that is certified by the appropriate state agency or agencies under regulations issued under Section 1616 (e) of the Social Security Act, which serves no more than 16 residents. (Office for Handicapped Individuals [OHI], 1980, Summary, p. 88)

Each otherwise eligible disabled person is to be treated as an "individual household" for purposes of determining eligibility and monthly coupon allotment. The term "food" was also redefined in the 1979 amendments to mean meals served in small group living arrangements. "Retail food store" was defined to include group living arrangements. Prior to the enactment of the 1979 amendments, group homes that provided meals to their residents were considered "institutions" and the residents were ineligible for food stamps.

Figure 80 illustrates the spending history for the entire Food Stamp Program. This program is often cited as an example of a rapidly escalating entitlement program.

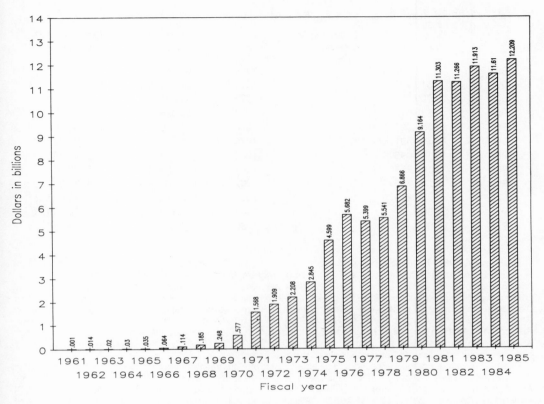

Figure 80.   Spending history of the Food Stamp Program: FY 1961–85.

In unadjusted terms, estimated Food Stamp Program spending for SSI recipients with mental retardation was $83.46 million in FY 1978 (see Table 40). Spending climbed steadily, doubling by FY 1981 to $169.63 million. This was an average annual growth rate of 27% between FY 1978 and FY 1981. By FY 1983, program assistance had advanced to $178.7 million. Spending in FY 1984, however, dropped by 2.5% to $174.15 million. The projection for FY 1985 was $183.14 million, an increase of 5% over the FY 1984 figure.

In real economic terms, the growth pattern averaged 15% annually between FY 1978 and FY 1981. It dipped by 9% in FY 1982, but increased slightly in FY 1983. The FY 1984 assistance figure dropped again—by 8%. Projected FY 1985 spending was virtually identical to the FY 1984 assistance level (see Figure 81).

Social Security Act, Title XVI, Section 1615: Rehabilitation

Section 1615 of the Social Security Act as Amended authorized federal reimbursements to state rehabilitation agencies for SSI recipients who, consequent to a rehabilitation experience, have engaged in substantial gainful activity for a period of 9 months. This provision, limiting Section 1615 to apply only to SSI recipients who have secured gainful employment status, has dramatically reduced participants in the program. Prior to 1981, and the enactment of the Omnibus Budget Reconciliation Act (OBRA), Section 1615 SSI reimbursements were authorized for SSI recipients regardless of rehabilitation outcome status.

The Social Security Act Amendments of 1976 authorized special provisions for SSI-eligible disabled children under age 16 years.

Table 40.   Food Stamp Program funding: FY 1961–85 (dollars are in thousands)

FY	Total program funding	Estimated MR payments	FY	Total program funding	Estimated MR payments
1961	$857		1974	$2,844,815	
1962	$13,700		1975	$4,598,956	
1963	$20,000		1976	$5,681,954	
1964	$30,015		1977	$5,398,795	
1965	$34,395		1978	$5,540,877	$83,458
1966	$64,491		1979	$6,866,287	$104,041
1967	$114,095		1980	$9,163,946	$137,785
1968	$184,727		1981	$11,303,025	$169,641
1969	$247,766		1982	$11,265,900	$168,988
1970	$576,810		1983	$11,913,000	$178,695
1971	$1,567,767		1984	$11,610,000	$174,150
1972	$1,909,166		1985	$12,209,000	$183,135
1973	$2,207,532				

Source: FY 1961–81 total program funding data are from Administrative Records, U.S. Department of Agriculture, Food and Nutrition Service, Food Stamp Program, Budget Office (G. Dyson, personal communication, September 18, 1983). The FY 1982–85 data are also from the Budget Office (S. Carlson, personal communication, November 15, 1984). To project an MR estimate, it was necessary to identify surveys indicating the degree to which SSI public assistance recipients with mental retardation were participating in the Food Stamp Program. According to the Food Stamp Program Budget Office (S. Carlson, personal communication, August 14, 1983), in August, 1981, 691,000 "blind and disabled" households were receiving an average assistance payment of $982 per year. Thus 691,000 × $982 = $678,562,000 in annual expenditures for the blind and disabled SSI recipient component of the SSI Program.

Twenty-five percent of the total blind and disabled SSI group are estimated to be mentally retarded, according to a utilization study described in this chapter's preceding entry on SSI (J. Schmulowitz, Social Security Administration, personal communication, June, 1983). Assuming equivalent rates of food stamp and cash SSI assistance utilization, 25% × $678,562,000 = $169,640,500 estimated food stamp assistance to persons with mental retardation in FY 1981. This represents 1.5% of all Food Stamp Program budget outlays that year. This assumption has been applied to annual Food Stamp Program assistance payments in the table.

The 1977 amendments to the Food Stamp Act enabled groups of SSI individuals to be certified as eligible for food stamps on the basis of SSI information in their files at Social Security offices. The Food Stamp Program Office (S. Carlson, personal communication, August 14, 1983) suggested that it was probably unlikely that large numbers of SSI clients with mental retardation came into the program until FY 1978 or later. Therefore, the earliest year for which an MR estimate is presented in the table is FY 1978.

These children must be referred to the state's Crippled Children agency. At least 90% of a state's allocation was required to be provided to children under 6, or to children who had never attended a public school. (Table 41 presents financial and client data for the rehabilitation program under Section 1615 as well as a similar program under Section 222 that is legislatively linked with the Social Security Trust fund discussed later in this chapter.

TRUST FUNDS

Social Security Act, Title II, Section 202(d): Adult Disabled Child Program

Benefit payments under the Adult Disabled Child (ADC) Program were originally autho-

rized under Section 202 (d) of the 1956 amendments to the Social Security Act. Section 202 (d) authorized payments to surviving disabled children aged 18 or older of retired, deceased, or disabled workers who are eligible to receive Social Security benefits. Dependent children (under age 18) of covered workers have received benefits since 1939, but not on the basis of their disability. Disability is defined under the act as an ". . . inability to engage in any substantial gainful activity by reason of any medically determinable physical or mental impairment which can be expected to last for a continuous period of not less than 12 months."

Figure 82 depicts the increasing number of beneficiaries with mental retardation in the ADC Program. It is noteworthy that it was

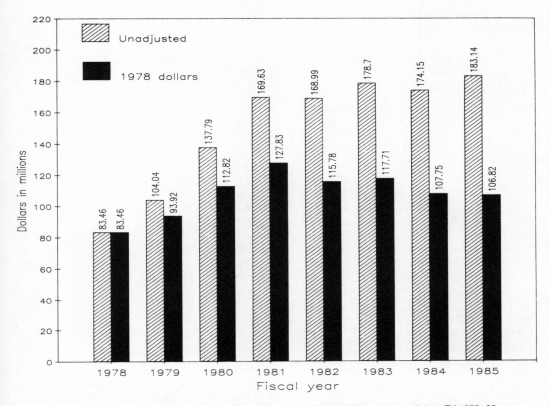

Figure 81. Estimated Food Stamp Program assistance to persons with mental retardation: FY 1978–85.

originally estimated prior to implementation of the program that there would only be about 20,000 eligible beneficiaries in the entire United States (Boggs, 1971). In 1984, ADC total enrollment reached 503,000, of whom about 362,000 were mentally retarded (see Table 42). Boggs (1971) commented that the unexpected experience of the Social Security Administration with the number of ADC beneficiaries "has demonstrated, as almost no other program could have done, the extent of disability due to mental retardation in the noninstitutionalized adult population" (p.111).

ADC benefit payments to persons with mental retardation have exhibited continuous and strong growth during FY 1957–85 on an unadjusted basis. Growth averaged an annual increment of 16% during the 1960s; 16% during the 1970s; and 11% during FY 1980–85. Projected total benefit payments for FY 1985 were 8% above the FY 1984 level. On an adjusted basis, the rate of growth is continuous, except for FY 1973; however, the growth rate slowed considerably during FY 1981–83. The average rate of growth in real economic terms was 11% for the 1960s (see Figure 83), and 8% for the 1970s (see Figure 84). For FY 1981–85, the rate of growth was 2.5% per annum.

During FY 1981–82, more than 400,000 disabled persons were informed that they would be removed from the disability rolls, although about 50% of those who appealed their decisions ultimately had their benefits restored. The great majority of those persons removed from the rolls were individuals with mental illness, chronic pain, or physical disabilities. Relatively few persons with mental retardation were affected; however, the rate of growth of beneficiaries with mental retardation in the ADC Program slowed appreciably in 1982.

Table 41. Section 1615 (SSI) and Section 222 (SSDI) rehabilitation funding: FY 1966–85 (dollars are in thousands)

FY	Total SSI expenditures	SSI clients	Total SSDI expenditures	SSDI beneficiaries	% MR clients rehabilitated	Estimated SSI-MR funds	Estimated SSDI-MR funds
1966			$468	NA	9.3%		$43
1967			$9,846	NA	10.2%		$1,004
1968			$15,440	26,455	10.7%		$1,652
1969			$17,557	32,911	11.4%		$2,001
1970			$20,983	35,275	11.8%		$2,475
1971			$24,375	40,711	12.5%		$3,046
1972			$30,390	45,111	11.6%		$3,525
1973	$6,862		$42,934	52,011	12.1%	$830	$5,195
1974	$11,395		$56,461	60,651	12.6%	$1,436	$7,114
1975	$47,782	38,232	$81,022	69,653	12.4%	$5,925	$10,047
1976	$52,721	53,924	$96,190	78,063	12.2%	$6,432	$11,735
1977	$48,479	47,602	$89,243	80,037	12.2%	$5,914	$10,888
1978	$50,925	55,218	$96,963	94,979	12.4%	$6,315	$12,023
1979	$53,999	57,897	$102,070	94,936	12.1%	$6,534	$12,350
1980	$55,000	52,000	$113,268	96,000	11.7%	$6,435	$13,252
1981	$37,000		$87,050		11.6%	$4,292	$10,097
1982	$1,043		$2,457		12.4%	$129	$305
1983	$2,982		$7,018		12.0%	$358	$842
1984	$2,982		$7,018		12.0%	$358	$842
1985	$3,700		$8,150		12.0%	$444	$978

Source: Data for FY 1966–81 are from U.S. Department of Education, Rehabilitation Services Administration, Administrative Records (S. Cohen, personal communication, November 15, 1984). Data provided for FY 1982–84 had combined SSDI-SSI amounts. The author apportioned the combined amounts according to the actual FY 1981 ratio between total expenditures for the SSDI and SSI rehabilitation programs. The OBRA of 1981 authorized the consolidation of SSI and SSDI rehabilitation funds. The total combined funding for these two programs under OBRA was: FY 1982, $3.5 million; FY 1983, $10 million; and FY 1984, $10 million. FY 1985 appropriation data were provided by the SSA, Office of Disability, Division of Vocational Rehabilitation and Special Programs (H. Allen, personal communication, November 21, 1984). Clients with mental retardation rehabilitated figures were obtained from Chapter 3 of this volume, Table 8.

Social Security Act, Title II, Section 222: Rehabilitation Program

Section 222 of the act required all applicants and recipients of Title II Disability Insurance benefits to be referred to the state vocational rehabilitation agency. Funds were authorized to be transferred from the Disability Insurance Trust Fund to state vocational rehabilitation agencies to reimburse the agencies for the provision of rehabilitation services to Title II applicants and beneficiaries. (Consult Table 41 for data on Section 222).

Section 222 authorized a 9-month "trial work period" for disabled Title II beneficiaries who are attempting to return to work. During this period, benefits are continued even though beneficiaries' monthly earnings may exceed the substantial gainful activity test. PL 96-265, the Social Security Disability Amendments of 1980, extended the trial work period to 24 months if a disabled beneficiary's earnings fell below the SGA test level during any month subsequent to termination of benefits at the end of a trial work period.

Table 42. Estimated Adult Disabled Child (ADC) Program benefits for FY 1957–85 (dollars are in thousands)

FY	Total beneficiaries	Estimated MR beneficiaries	Total benefits	MR benefits
1957	28,869	19,660	$13,380	$9,112
1958	47,025	32,024	$22,356	$15,224
1959	82,453	56,150	$42,504	$28,945
1960	104,054	70,861	$55,128	$37,542
1961	124,221	84,595	$68,753	$46,821
1962	147,264	100,287	$82,378	$56,099
1963	166,642	113,483	$96,003	$65,378
1964	183,522	124,978	$109,628	$74,657
1965	198,390	135,104	$123,252	$83,935
1966	213,721	145,544	$134,448	$91,559
1967	229,658	156,397	$147,180	$100,230
1968	243,654	165,928	$180,780	$123,111
1969	257,222	175,168	$193,824	$131,994
1970	270,557	188,308	$237,684	$165,428
1971	285,061	198,402	$278,952	$194,151
1972	305,007	212,285	$361,668	$251,721
1973	319,988	222,712	$384,516	$267,623
1974	341,082	237,393	$460,236	$320,324
1975	362,335	252,185	$533,940	$371,622
1976	381,563	265,568	$605,856	$421,676
1977	404,246	281,355	$689,436	$479,847
1978	419,896	292,248	$774,240	$538,871
1979	435,338	302,995	$896,172	$623,736
1980	450,169	313,318	$1,075,704	$748,690
1981	463,021	333,375	$1,247,412	$898,137
1982	472,416	340,140	$1,389,276	$1,000,279
1983	488,372	351,628	$1,510,728	$1,087,724
1984	503,000	362,160	$1,635,000	$1,177,200
1985	517,000	372,240	$1,768,000	$1,272,960

Source: Primary documents from which prevalence statistics and payment amounts for FY 1957–83 were obtained include the "Social Security Bulletin, Annual Statistical Supplement" for 1981 (U.S. Department of Health and Human Services, 1981, Table 100) and the "Annual Statistical Supplement" for 1983 (DHHS, 1983, Table 87). Payment data and recipient figures for FY 1984 and FY 1985 were provided by Jeff Kunkel, SSA, Office of the Actuary (personal communication, December 11, 1984). Kay Allen, Bob Cormier, and Phil Lerner, SSA, Office of Research and Statistics also provided guidance (personal communications, August, 1983). Total estimated Adult Disabled Child benefits for FY 1983–85 were provided by Lerner (personal communication, February, 1985) and include a cost-of-living increase and an increment for program growth predicated on demographics. The percentage of beneficiaries with mental retardation in the ADC Program from FY 1957 to FY 1969 was 68.1%, based on allowances during FY 1957–63 for individuals diagnosed as "mentally deficient," or mentally deficient in conjunction with a diagnosis of "cerebral spastic infantile paralysis" or "epilepsy" (Surveys and Research Corporation, 1965). The percentage of beneficiaries with mental retardation in the ADC program in 1970 was identified as 69.6%, according to an adult characteristics study published by the Social Security Administration (Braddock, 1973). In the absence of definitive information, the calculations of MR benefit payment levels during FY 1971–80 were predicated on the 1970 study prevalence rate. The Social Security Administration's Office of Disability Studies recommended increasing the MR participation rate to 72% during the 1981–85 period. This increase was based on a slight increase in the number of persons with mental retardation appearing on other federal benefit rolls such as SSI. The computation of annual MR benefit payment levels was achieved by multiplying the percentage of persons with mental retardation served in a given year times the total overall benefits paid to all disabled participants in the ADC Program.

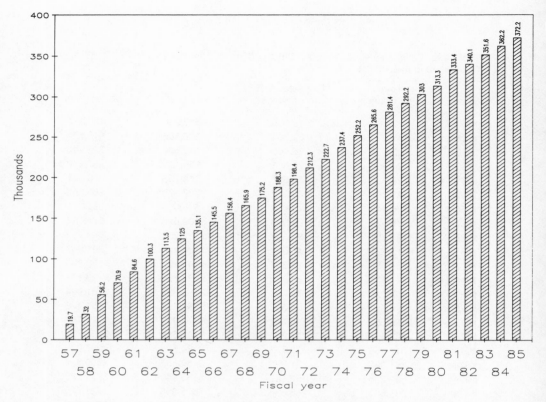

Figure 82.   Estimated beneficiaries with mental retardation in the ADC Program: FY 1957–85.

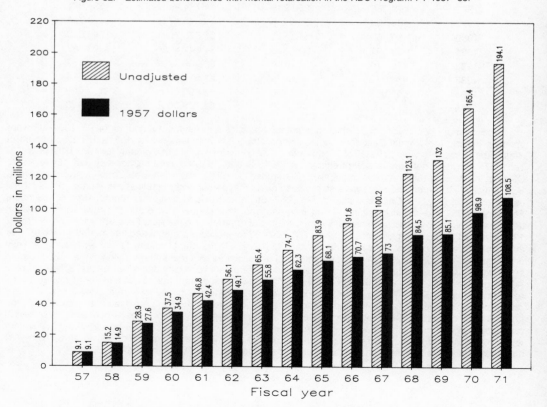

Figure 83.   Estimated ADC benefits paid to persons with mental retardation: FY 1957–71.

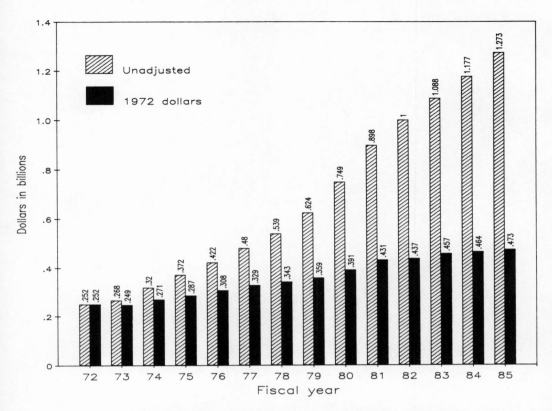

Figure 84.   Estimated ADC benefits paid to persons with mental retardation: FY 1972–85.

Chapter 7

Construction Programs

THE FEDERAL GOVERNMENT'S involvement in the construction of facilities for persons with mental disabilities began in 1933, with the passage of the National Industrial Recovery Act. Enacted during the depths of the Great Depression, this law authorized grants and loans for the construction of public buildings. State mental institutions received perhaps as much as $160 million in assistance during FY 1935–40. After the Second World War, the federal government undertook a systematic program of Surplus Property Disposal, initially authorized by law in 1944. Many schools for retarded persons and, in several cases, even entire state institutions were converted from previous use as a military institution or hospital. The cumulative market value of property transferring to MR/DD use is $28.31 million, as of FY 1985.

The modern era of federal health care construction grants began with the Hospital Survey and Construction Act, also known as the Hill-Burton Program. MR/DD facilities began receiving Hill-Burton assistance in FY 1958, and $32 million in federal construction grants were deployed to state institutions and nonprofit community facilities between FY 1957 and FY 1971.

In 1963, Congress enacted the Mental Retardation Facilities and Community Mental Health Centers Construction Act, PL 88-164. Title I of the act was the first specific federal construction legislation dedicated exclusively to the construction of mental health facilities. Implementation brought about the obligations of $155.8 million in federal funds over the next decade for Mental Retardation Research

Centers ($27 million), University Affiliated Facilities ($38.6 million), and Community Facilities ($90.2 million). An additional $5.1 million in construction funding were expended during FY 1972–76 under provisions of the Developmental Disabilities Services and Facilities Construction Act of 1970 (DD Act; PL 91-517).

More recently, PL 95-557, the 1978 Housing and Community Development Amendments, stipulated that a minimum of $50 million in U.S. Department of Housing and Urban Development (HUD) Section 202 construction loans be earmarked annually for nonelderly handicapped persons. Thus far, loan commitments have far exceeded that earmark ($96.1 million in FY 1985). Persons with MR/DD have participated extensively in the program, which is coordinated with the HUD Section Eight Rental Assistance Program. The Small Business Administration (SBA) has also been administering a loan program since FY 1974, in which MR/DD involvement is known to be an active component. An unknown but significant portion of the SBA loans are deployed for construction purposes.

The historical trends in construction funding seem to differ markedly from the rapid escalation in total funding that characterizes the federal mission in the provision of services. In fact, exclusive of Medicaid ICF/MR reimbursements to public and private MR/DD facilities, the federal government currently makes no grants for explicit MR/DD construction purposes. It has not done so since FY 1976, the year funds under the DD Act (PL 91-517) could no longer be used for construc-

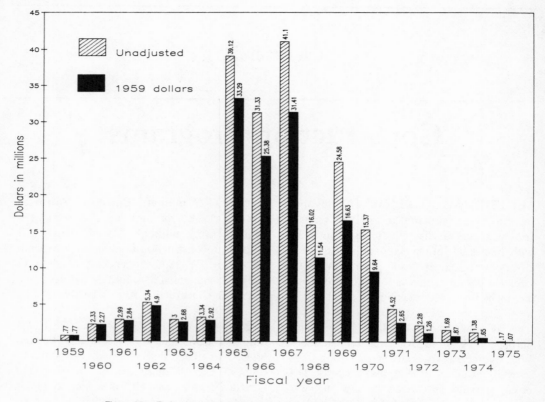

Figure 85.   Federal grants for the construction of MR/DD facilities: FY 1959–75.

tion. As shown in Figure 85, federal MR/DD construction grant funding has declined rapidly after its FY 1967 peak of $41.1 million.

The figure, however, omits federal construction reimbursements under the $2.66 billion ICF/MR Program and also Surplus Property Transfers. A national estimate is not available on the ICF/MR cost component attributable to federal ICF/MR reimbursements for construction amortization. However, a figure of $100 million annually during FY 1980–85, only 3.8% of total projected FY 1985 reimbursements, is probably not excessive, in view of the extensive renovation and construction activities going on in state institutions, and the fact that private ICFs/MR are also reimbursed for amortization of capital expenditures. Gettings and Mitchell (1980), for example, identified cumulative state-federal

MR/DD construction spending of nearly $1 billion between FY 1977 and FY 1979, much of which they attributed to ICF/MR-related activity.

The Surplus Property Disposal Program assigns a specific market value to transferred property. These figures can be used to index annual "spending" under the program. The value of transfers peaked in FY 1966–67 at $6 million, and since FY 1975 has never risen above $1 million per annum.

NATIONAL INDUSTRIAL RECOVERY ACT OF 1933: GRANTS AND LOANS

Between FY 1933 and FY 1937, during the Great Depression, the Public Works Administration was responsible for transacting $3.356 billion in federal construction grants and loans throughout the United States under the National Industrial Recovery Act Program (Short & Stanley-Brown, 1939). Projects completed included 718 new school buildings and 62 hospital and institutional projects. The program also resulted in the construction of the Washington Monument, the Federal Trade Commission building, the U.S. Mint, numerous ships, and public housing. Coliseums and exposition halls were built in many major cities and libraries were built for universities and towns throughout the United States. Fire and police stations, courthouses, one state supreme court building, and one state capitol (Oregon's) were also constructed. In addition, recreation and social buildings, bridges, highways, water treatment plants, sewage facilities, the Boulder and Grand Coulee Dams, and several zoos were erected.

Grants paid for up to 45% of all nonfederal project costs; loans at 4% interest were made for up to 55% of non-federal projects. About half of the $3.356 billion was directly administered by state and local governments. In total, there were a staggering 26,474 projects assisted, of which 8,259 were building projects. A total of 17,300 separate buildings were erected. (These figures reflect appropriations only through FY 1937. An additional 7,993 projects, including 10,350 buildings, had been completed or were under construction from the FY 1938 appropriation.)

Short and Stanley-Brown (1939) selected 620 architecturally representative projects, about 8% of those initiated between FY 1933 and FY 1937, and described them in detail. These descriptions were evaluated individually to identify grant and loan activities pertaining to handicapped persons. Short and Stanley-Brown (1939) noted in their foreword that "throughout the country, hospitals and state institutions have been able to build or greatly improve their plants for the insane, the sick, the aged, and the crippled" (p. xv).

Short and Stanley-Brown (1939) identified 62 hospital-institutional projects. Two pertained to MR/DD institutions. The administration building at the Fernald State School in Massachusetts was constructed in 1936, at a

Table 43.　Sampling of NIRA grants and loans for mental institution construction: FY 1933–39 (dollars are in thousands)

FY	Mental hospital funds	MR/DD Institution funds	Total funds
1933			$0
1934			$0
1935	$317		$317
1936	$990	$236	$1,226
1937	$5,049		$5,049
1938	$6,613		$6,613
1939	$3,269		$3,269
Total	$16,238	$236	$16,474

Source: Based on analysis of the data presented in Short and Stanley-Brown (1939). Funds in the table reflect funding for only a small number (8%) of the projects funded nationwide between FY 1933 and FY 1939. Numbers in the table should probably be multiplied several times to obtain an accurate picture of program funding.

cost of $112,000; and a dormitory was constructed at the "Epileptic Colony" in Sykesville, Maryland, at a cost of $124,626. However, large numbers of persons with mental retardation have historically resided in state mental hospitals; the Short and Stanley-Brown review identified 14 such projects in these settings. (See Table 43 for NIRA grants and loans used for mental institution construction.)

The list of mental hospitals assisted included: Pilgrim (New York, $2.5 million); Cranston (Rhode Island, $5.8 million); Ohio, 7 institutions, $874,000; Chicago State Hospital (Illinois, $5.7 million); Green Bay County Asylum (Wisconsin, $317,000); South Carolina State Hospital ($718,000); St. Joseph State Hospital (Missouri, $651,000); Moose Lake State Hospital (Minnesota, $2.4 million); Jameston State Hospital (North Dakota, $321,000); Pueblo State Hospital (Colorado, $424,000); Camarillo State Hospital (California, $670,000); Phoenix State Hospital (Arizona, $112,000 and $89,000); and Chatahoochie State Hospital (Florida, $118,000 and $358,000). Two institutions for blind persons, seven tuberculosis hospitals and the National Leprosarium, at Carsville, Louisiana, also received federal construction assistance.

SURPLUS PROPERTY ACT
OF 1944 AS AMENDED

The Office of Surplus Property Utilization, Office of Facilities Engineering and Property Management, within the Office of the Assistant Secretary for Administration and Management, U.S. Department of Health and Human Services (DHHS), carries out the responsibilities of the department under the Federal Property and Administrative Services Act of 1944 as Amended, which makes surplus federal real and personal properties available for health and educational purposes. The properties that become available under this program are those that have been determined by the General Services Administration (GSA) as having no further federal utilization. The 1944 act was revised and superseded by the Surplus Property Act of 1949 as Amended.

Surplus personal properties generated at federal installations in the United States, Europe, and Southeast Asia are screened to determine those that may be needed and may be usable in health and educational programs. Properties determined to have utility are allocated by the DHHS and the Department of Education for transfer to state agencies for surplus property.

An applicant for real property must be a state, or a political subdivision or instrumentality thereof; a tax-supported educational or public health institution; or a nonprofit educational or public health institution that has been held to be exempt from taxation under Section 501 (c)(3) of the Internal Revenue Code of 1954. Its proposed program of use must be fundamentally for an educational or public health purpose (i.e., devoted to academic, vocational, or professional instruction, or organized and operated to promote and protect the public health). Real property may be put to joint use, namely for the training of persons with MR/DD as well as persons with physical handicaps.

Because most federal property was transferred prior to the relatively recent movement to fully integrate disabled persons into education, health, and human services programs, most property transfer applications implicitly encouraged the provision of services to persons with mental retardation in segregated settings. However, no recent property transfers have been designated for use by the states as institutions.

Georgia established a 400–800 bed rehabilitation facility for persons with mental disabilities on the former Veterans Administration (VA) Domiciliary, in Thomasville and, in 1974, acquired another 18-acre portion as the site for the care of alcoholics, and persons with mental retardation and other handicaps. The state has also established a Regional Mental Hospital at the former U.S. Penitentiary Honor Farm near Atlanta, and the Augusta Association for Retarded Citizens acquired three buildings at Fort Gordon for removal to a new site for the care of persons with mental retardation.

Many other states operate similar institutions, such as: the Sunland Training Center, located at former Graham Air Force Station, Florida; the New York State Hospital, operating at the former VA Hospital at Tupper Lake; Ohio's Broadview Center for the Mentally Retarded near Columbia; Lufkin State Hospital in Texas; Kansas Neurological Institute, at the former VA Winter Hospital, Topeka; and the Illinois Fox Developmental Center at Dwight, formerly the Dwight VA Hospital.

Many programs are operated by entities other than states, such as counties, local school boards, and associations for retarded citizens. In 1974, for example, the Eastern Idaho Child Development Center acquired a portion of the Victor Ranger Station to use for the education of handicapped persons. Lake Charles Association for Retarded Citizens, Louisiana, received 8 acres and a building at Chennault Air Force Base. In Kentucky, 3.2 acres and two buildings at the former Ranger Headquarters in Williamsburg were conveyed to the Whiteley County Board of Education for classrooms and a playground for the children; .38 acre was conveyed to Cumberland River Regional Mental Health Center as the site for a school for children with mental retardation. Melwood Horticultural Training Center in Maryland acquired the former Federal Broadcast Information Station at Oxon Hill for training retarded persons in horticulture. In

Montana, the Opportunity School Foundation acquired 5 acres at the Forest Service site at Fort Missoula.

The record of the House appropriations hearings on the proposed FY 1977 Department of Health, Education and Welfare (HEW) budget indicated that through June 30, 1974, 5,411 acres of land and 894 buildings had been transferred for use in programs serving persons with MR/DD (Office for Handicapped Individuals [OHI], 1976). These properties originally cost the federal government $49.4 million and had a fair market value of $20.7 million (OHI, 1976). Most of the property ($31 million) was transferred between FY 1964 and FY 1974.

When a property is transferred, the associated administrative procedures typically require the recording of the "acquisition cost," the price the U.S. government paid for the property, and the "fair market value," (what the property is actually worth at the time the transfer is made). The recipient is then required to dedicate the property to the use agreed upon for a specific number of years. Since fair market value is a more accurate reflection of the economic value of the new asset at the time the actual transaction between the federal government and the recipients takes place, it was used to measure the intensity of federal allocations over the 40-year history of the program. In unadjusted terms, the aggregate fair market value of all property transferred between FY 1947 and FY 1985 was $28.3 million (see Table 44). Property put to mental retardation use was transferred first in FY 1947, not at all during FY 1948–54 and FY 1956, and continuously since FY 1957. Through FY 1958, the median asset value of annual transfers was only $31,000. From FY 1959 to FY 1963, the median value rose to $669,000. The program reached peak allocation levels during FY 1964–67, when a combined total of $15 million in property was transferred. More than one-half of the program's property transfers for MR/DD use was conveyed during that period.

Allocations declined from FY 1968 to FY 1976, to a median value of $765,000. For FY 1978–80, annual transfer values dipped to a median figure of $149,000. The FY 1981–84

Table 44.   Cost/value of MR/DD surplus property transferred: FY 1947–85

FY	Acquisition cost	Fair market value
1947	$230,127	$45,000
1955	$303,206	$92,000
1957	$10,494	$8,750
1958	$23,002	$16,100
1959	$5,382,892	$799,778
1960	$160,223	$109,250
1961	$9,271,592	$778,439
1962	$496,169	$554,600
1963	$535,247	$668,480
1964	$4,163,109	$2,202,004
1965	$97,092	$90,100
1966	$9,671,882	$6,412,884
1967	$10,212,915	$6,238,121
1968	$3,043,191	$929,500
1969	$874,245	$270,772
1970	$208,710	$319,300
1971	$8,653,425	$1,309,300
1972	$2,361,733	$764,710
1973	$559,376	$328,218
1974	$4,626,900	$855,548
1975	$2,690,650	$1,000,445
1976	$1,047,515	$964,934
1977	$570,753	$233,410
1978	$73,413	$27,285
1979	$518,232	$191,745
1980	$285,200	$105,524
1981	$1,121,018	$414,776
1982	$3,956,781	$647,000
1983	$3,039,720	$622,000
1984	$3,139,720	$714,000
1985(e)[a]	$2,814,309	$599,000
Total	$80,142,841	$28,312,973

Source: Administrative Records were provided by the DHHS, Office of the Assistant Secretary for Management and Budget, Office of Facilities Engineering, Office of Real Property, Division of Realty (L. Sparklin, realty specialist, personal communications, November 29, 1983, and November 28, 1984). The records documented transfers of property from the War Assets Administration authorized by the 1944 act, including all MR/DD property transferred by the Federal Security Agency and the Department of Health, Education, and Welfare (DHEW). These records were inspected by the author and included as appropriate. It should be noted that after PL 96-88 established the U.S. Department of Education, administrative responsibility for cases involving educational property was transferred to the Department of Education. Data on Department of Education transfers for FY 1982–85 were obtained through the Department of Education, Regional Liaison Unit (A. Kelly, personal communication, December 6, 1984). Figures for FY 1985 are estimates based on the average of the previous 4 years of data.

[a]Estimated.

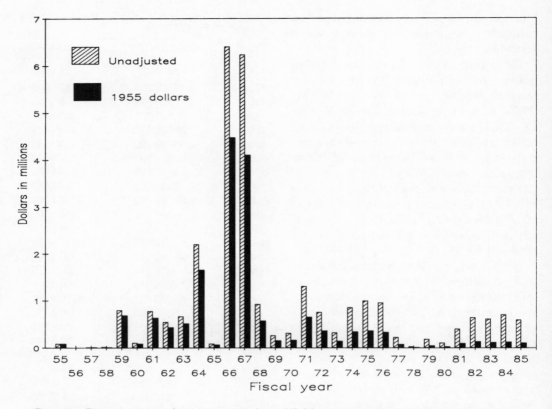

Figure 86.   Fair market values of real property transfers to MR/DD use under the Surplus Property Act as Amended:
FY 1955–85.

median figure increased to $622,000. These trends are displayed in Figure 86.

In January, 1983, President Ronald Reagan issued Executive Order 12348 establishing the Federal Property Review Board. The board's purpose was to identify surplus property and market it for sale, thus increasing revenues. The board initially was headed by former White House staff member Edwin Meese, and it included among its membership the GSA administrator.

HILL-BURTON CONSTRUCTION ACT MEDICAL FACILITIES CONSTRUCTION

The Hill-Burton Construction Act, originally enacted in 1946, authorized the nation's first systematic grant program specifically devoted to hospital construction. Previous federal public health construction assistance had been tied

to general Public Works Administration projects authorized during the Depression under the National Industrial Recovery Act and, to "impact aid" for hospital construction projects in communities affected by defense-related population increases during World War II.

The purpose of the Hill-Burton Act was to make available "adequate hospitals, clinics, and similar services to all people." Initially, a special priority was placed on supporting general hospital construction in communities with the greatest need, especially rural areas. The federal-state/local matching percentage was 25%:75% under the original act; however, due to amendments in 1949, the match was changed to allow a sliding scale federal share of 25% to 75%, depending on state needs and the economic status of the community. The

1949 amendments also doubled the program's authorization level from $75 million to $150 million.

The deployment of Hill-Burton funds for any hospital furnishing primarily domiciliary care was prohibited by Public Health Services regulation. Until FY 1958, funds were not available to the states for construction projects at mental retardation institutions. Remarkably, this policy was in force even though Senator Lister Hill clearly stated in a 1954 letter to the National Association for Retarded Children (NARC) that he, a co-sponsor of the legislation, "had no intention of making such an exclusion of treatment facilities for any groups. . ." (Boggs, 1971, p.111).

Between FY 1958 and FY 1964, however, Hill-Burton was an important source of construction funds for mental retardation projects at state institutions, activity centers, and

workshops throughout the country. Until the passage of the Mental Retardation Facilities and Community Mental Health Centers Act in 1963, the Hill-Burton Program was the primary source of federal assistance for mental retardation construction. Mental retardation facilities began receiving construction and consultation assistance in FY 1958. State mental retardation institutions, day care centers, workshops, and various nonprofit facilities serving persons with mental retardation received 90 awards and $32 million in federal aid between FY 1958 and FY 1971 (Braddock, 1973, p.131). In any single year, total mental retardation construction spending never exceeded 3.3% of total Hill-Burton Act expenditures. (See Table 45 for annual mental retardation construction funds expended.)

Hill-Burton support peaked in FY 1965 at $6.5 million, but plunged during FY 1967–69

Table 45. MR/DD construction expenditures: FY 1958–76 (dollars are in thousands)

FY	PL 88-164 Part A: Research Centers	PL 88-164 Part B: UAFs	PL 88-164 Part C: Community Facilities	PL 91-517 Formula Grants	Hill-Burton Act
1958					$43
1959					$774
1960					$2,329
1961					$2,989
1962					$5,338
1963					$2,996
1964					$3,340
1965	$14,745	$7,223	$10,700		$6,455
1966	$6,234	$7,021	$15,641		$2,319
1967	$6,026	$16,105	$18,276		$235
1968		$0	$14,757		$973
1969		$6,600	$16,854		$739
1970		$0	$14,013		$1,086
1971		$1,591			$2,395
1972		$0		$1,796	
1973		$31		$1,584	
1974				$1,380	
1975				$172	
1976				$172	
Totals	$27,005	$38,571	$90,241	$5,104	$31,968

Source: All fiscal data pertinent to PL 88-164, Parts A, B, and C, were obtained from Braddock (1973, p. 137), except UAF data for Part B in 1973, which were obtained from FY 1975 House hearings (Office of Mental Retardation Coordination [OMRC], 1974, p. 62).

Data presented on PL 91-517 were reported by the DHHS in various annual House appropriation hearings. FY 1972 data are from FY 1974 hearings (Office of Mental Retardation Coordination [OMRC], 1973, p. 65); FY 1973 data are from FY 1975 hearings (OMRC, 1974, p. 62); FY 1974–76 data are from FY 1976 hearings (Office for Handicapped Individuals [OHI], 1975, p. 68). The source of Hill-Burton figures is Braddock (1973, p. 131).

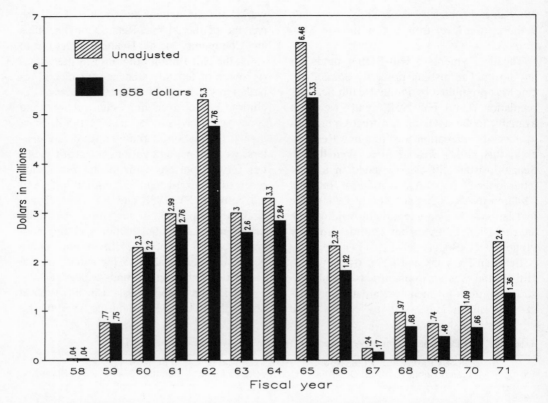

Figure 87.   Construction spending under the Hill-Burton Act for mental retardation facilities: FY 1958–71.

to a median level of $739,000. In FY 1970–71, the funding level was $1.1 and $2.4 million, respectively. Mental retardation support was terminated in FY 1971. Figure 87 illustrates this history.

PL 88-164: MENTAL RETARDATION FACILITIES AND COMMUNITY MENTAL HEALTH CENTERS CONSTRUCTION ACT

Enacted in 1963, and embodying several recommendations of the President's Panel on Mental Retardation (1962), PL 88-164 comprised three interrelated construction programs. Part A authorized the construction of the Mental Retardation Research Centers, Part B authorized construction support for University Affiliated Facilities (UAFs), and Part C authorized the construction of Community Facilities.

PL 90-170, the mental retardation amendments of 1967, extended and expanded, through June 30, 1970, the construction authorities supporting Parts B and C, and added a new Part D which authorized systematically declining matching staffing grants for community mental retardation facilities. In 1970, the Developmental Disabilities Services and Facilities Construction Act (PL 91-517) extended the construction authority for Parts B and C until June 30, 1973.

Title I, Part A of PL 88-164 authorized construction grants for facilities in which medical and behavioral research relating to human development would be conducted to assist in the prevention and amelioration of mental retardation. Twelve centers received funds for construction; however, the Joseph P. Kennedy Foundation contributed the 25% nonfederal match for several of them.

The 12 research centers presently receiving funds include the Universities of California (at Los Angeles and San Francisco), Yeshiva, Washington, Kansas, Vanderbilt, North Carolina, Wisconsin, Colorado, and Chicago, and the Children's Hospital Corporation in Boston and the Eunice K. Shriver Center for Mental Retardation, Inc. in Waltham, Massachusetts. The Research Centers Program is currently administered by the mental retardation branch of the National Institute of Child Health and Human Development (NICHD). Federal construction funds for the centers were deployed in FY 1965–67. Funding was $14.75 million in FY 1965; $6.2 million in FY 1966; and $6.03 million in FY 1967 (see Table 45).

Title I, Part B of the 1963 act authorized project grants to assist in the construction of public or nonprofit clinical facilities for persons with mental retardation that were associated with a college or university. These UAFs were authorized to demonstrate specialized services for mental retardation diagnosis and treatment and to aid in the clinical training of physicians and other specialized personnel. Eighteen UAFs had received federal funds for construction as of December 31, 1970. One UAF was constructed with monies available under Title I, Part A. In late 1984, 43 UAFs and satellites were receiving core operational support from the federal government's Administration on Developmental Disabilities (ADD). ADD was also negotiating several new satellite awards for FY 1985 funding.

The original construction grants for UAFs were made over a 9-year period, FY 1965–73. In total, $38.6 million was budgeted for UAF construction. The annual obligations were: $7.22 million in FY 1965; $7.02 million in FY 1966; $16.1 million in FY 1967; $6.6 million in FY 1969; $1.6 million in FY 1971; and $31,000 in FY 1973 (see Table 45).

The Community Facilities Construction Program, authorized under Title I, Part C, provided federal grants to states to assist in the construction of specially designed public or other nonprofit facilities for the diagnosis, treatment, education, training, and personal care of persons with MR/DD. This program was modeled after the Hill-Burton Act hospital construction program.

A total of 362 projects were funded for $90.2 million between FY 1965 and FY 1970

(see Table 45). This figure includes $21.38 million appropriated pursuant to Title II of PL 88-164 for mental health facility construction, but actually obligated under Title I for mental retardation community facility construction; and $1.37 million appropriated pursuant to Title I, but obligated under Title II of the act for mental health expenditures.

Figure 88 displays aggregate annual construction funding for research centers, UAFs, and community facilities. Total funding for all construction activity over the entire funding history of the program, between FY 1965 and FY 1973, was $155.817 million.

The mental retardation amendments of 1967, PL 90-170, extended through June 30, 1970, the construction authorities supporting UAF and community facility construction. It also added a new Part D, authorizing federal staffing grants for the community facilities. In 1970, the Developmental Disabilities Services and Facilities Construction Act, PL 91-517, extended the construction authority for Parts B and C until June 30, 1973.

PL 91-517 (DD ACT): FORMULA GRANT CONSTRUCTION

PL 91-517 authorized a program of state formula grants. The states were given the authority to expend the funds for planning, services, administration, and construction. A few states between FY 1972 and FY 1976 opted to spend a small portion of their state funds for construction. Sums expended for construction during this period under the act can be found in Table 45.

PL 89-333, SECTION 12: REHABILITATION GRANTS

In 1966, PL 89-333 amended the Vocational Rehabilitation Act by authorizing project grants to assist in meeting the construction costs of public and other nonprofit rehabilitation facilities. Between FY 1966 and FY 1973, $22.765 million in federal funds was obligated for Section 12 grants by the Rehabilitation Services Administration (see Table 46). Precise data, however, were not available on the extent

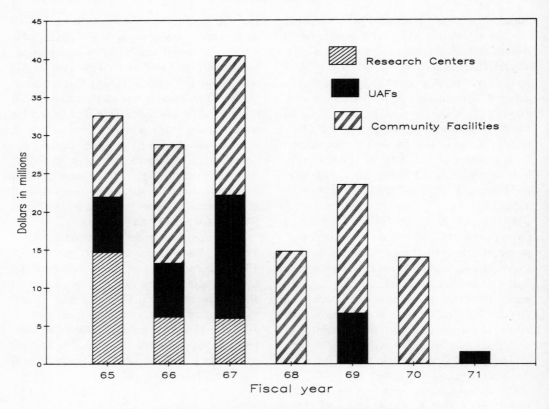

Figure 88.   Construction expenditures under PL 88-164: FY 1965–71.

Table 46.   Rehabilitation facility construction grants funded under Section 12: FY 1966–73 (dollars are in thousands)

FY	Total Section 12 funds	% MR clients rehabilitated	Estimated MR funds
1966	$1,500	9.3%	$140
1967	$4,500	10.2%	$459
1968	$2,669	10.5%	$286
1969	$3,383	11.4%	$386
1970	$2,274	11.8%	$268
1971	$4,240	12.5%	$530
1972	$3,649	11.6%	$489
1973	$550	12.1%	$77

Source: Braddock (1973, p. 96). Estimated mental retardation funds are based on the percentage of clients rehabilitated under the state-federal Vocational Rehabilitation Grant Program (see Table 8 of this book).

to which these construction funds assisted in the provision of services to individuals with mental retardation. However, many of the grants were made to build sheltered workshops and other community-based rehabilitation facilities known to serve persons with mental retardation.

SECTION 202: HOUSING LOANS

Section 202 of the Housing Act of 1959 (PL 86-372) originated as a program of direct loans to aid local nonprofit agencies in the provision of housing for elderly individuals. The Housing Act of 1964 (PL 88-560) amended Section 202 to extend housing loans to projects for physically handicapped persons as well. The Housing and Community Development Act of 1974, PL 93-383, substantially improved the subsidy mechanism and broadened the target population to encompass both physically and mentally handicapped persons. Individuals with MR/DD were explicitly included in the amended statutory definition of "low income families." PL 95-128, the Housing and Community Development Act of 1977, mandated coordination of applications for Section 202 loans and Section 8 rental assistance payments.

The 1978 housing amendments, PL 95-557, mandated that a minimum of $50 million in FY 1979 Section 202 loan funds be set aside for the construction and rehabilitation of housing for "non-elderly handicapped persons." (Elderly handicapped persons are eligible on the basis of their advanced age rather than their handicap.) The statutory purpose of these funds was to: 1) support innovative methods of meeting the needs of handicapped persons by providing a variety of housing options ranging from small group homes to independent living complexes, 2) provide handicapped occupants with a range of services and opportunities for independent living and participation in normal daily activities, and 3) facilitate the access of handicapped persons to general community activities and to suitable employment within the community.

Under Section 202, the term "handicapped persons" is defined as persons having an impairment that is expected to be of long, continuing, and indefinite duration. It must substantially impede one's ability to live indepen-

Table 47. Section 202 loans: FY 1976–85 (dollars are in thousands)

FY	MR/DD loans approved	# of MR/DD projects	Total Section 202 units	Total Section 202 elderly and handicapped loans
1976	$699	1	26,400	$632,000
1977	$1,117	1	21,000	$637,000
1978	$6,898	12	19,200	$629,700
1979	$4,265	14	20,000	$726,000
1980	$35,263	73	17,900	$687,000
1981	$44,287	86	14,470	$687,000
1982	$40,852	68	15,525	$716,000
1983	$37,298	(1,006 units) 69	13,300	$536,000
1984	$50,668	(1,349 units) 107	14,024	$604,000
1985	$50,332			$600,000

FY	Handicapped loans	% Handicapped	Handicapped units
1976			
1977			
1978	$67,400	11%	2,300
1979	$74,200	10%	2,217
1980	$63,200	9%	1,900
1981	$70,100	10%	1,613
1982	$87,000	12%	2,048
1983	$59,000	11%	1,600
1984	$96,766	16%	2,499
1985	$96,125	16%	

Source: Section 202 loan data for FY 1976–85 are from the HUD Office of Management Information Systems, Direct Loan Branch (S. Falconer, personal communications, October 25, 1983, and December 4, 1984). The FY 1985 MR/DD loan figure is an estimate based on the total Section 202 FY 1985 appropriation. The total appropriation decreased by .66% ($4 million) in FY 1985, so the author decreased the FY 1984 MR/DD loan figure by that same amount.

dently, and it must be of a nature such that that ability could be improved by more suitable housing conditions. The definition specifically includes individuals with MR/DD. Handicapped "families" eligible to live in Section 202 projects may include two or more handicapped persons living together; or one or more handicapped persons living with another person who is determined to be essential to his or her care or well being. In addition to building or renovating basic housing units, Section 202 Direct Loans may be used for certain related structures designed to meet the specialized needs of handicapped persons.

In FY 1984, over 50% of the total number of Section 202–sponsored nonelderly handicapped units were apartments or group homes specifically for individuals with MR/DD. Eligible applicants for Section 202 loans may borrow from HUD up to 100% of the total development cost of the projects. Loans may be repaid over a 40-year period at an interest

rate based on the average rate paid by the U.S. Treasury in its borrowing activities.

The volume of approved loans for MR/DD purposes increased rapidly from FY 1976 to FY 1981, advancing on an unadjusted basis from $699,000 to $44.3 million (see Table 47). Approvals dipped during FY 1982–83 to $40.9 million and $37.3 million, respectively. The FY 1984 approval rate established a new peak of $50.7 million.

In real economic terms, approved MR/DD loans also exhibited a strong upward trend through FY 1981, but plunged by a factor of 6.2% in FY 1982 and 11.5% in FY 1983. In FY 1984, loans surged to an amount approximately equivalent to their FY 1981 level. Figure 89 illustrates these trends.

During FY 1976–85, a total of 431 project proposals in developmental disabilities were approved. These trends are illustrated in Figure 90.

The developmental disabilities field has

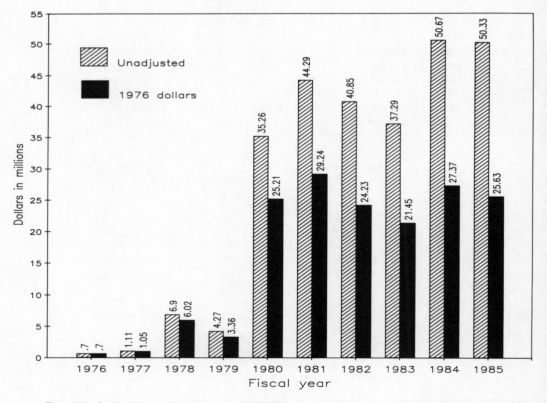

Figure 89.   Section 202 loan funds approved for MR/DD construction and renovation projects: FY 1976–85.

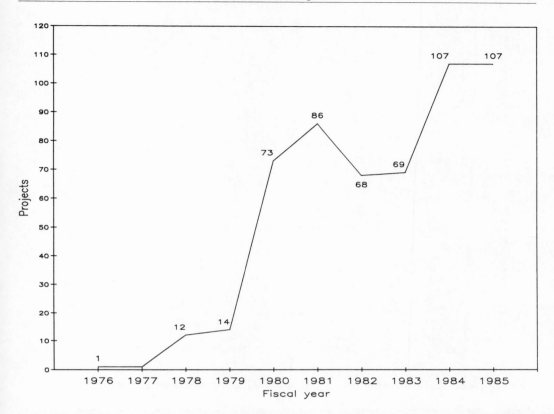

Figure 90. MR/DD loan projects approved under the Section 202 construction and renovation program: FY 1976–85.

been particularly effective in obtaining its share of funds in the Handicapped Loan Program. Since FY 1980, the annual percentage of MR/DD loans among all funds approved for the Handicapped program failed to exceed 50% only in FY 1982, when the rate fell to 47% from 63% the year before (see Figure 91).

The trend in total appropriations for the entire Section 202 Elderly and Handicapped Loan Program has been inconsistent from year to year. The dominant pattern is relatively stable in unadjusted terms, particularly if the FY 1979 peak of $726 million and the FY 1983 bottom of $536 million are excluded. The average annual appropriation during FY 1976–85 was $645 million. In real economic terms, however, appropriations have plunged dramatically from earlier levels. The FY 1985 appropriation is 52% less than the FY 1976 peak figure. Real year-to-year appropriations

diminished every year during the FY 1976–85 span, except in FY 1979 and FY 1984, when funding rose by 4% and 5.8%, respectively. Trends in total funding for the Elderly and Handicapped Loan Program are illustrated in Figure 92. In view of this substantial slide in real funding for the Elderly and Handicapped Loan Program, commitments for MR/DD projects have been remarkably vigorous.

Loans for handicapped projects in general have exhibited increased strength since FY 1980, constituting 9.2% of total Section 202 elderly and handicapped loans in that year, 10% in FY 1981, 12% the following year, 11% in FY 1983, and 16% in FY 1984–85. Loan approval levels for the Handicapped Program were fairly stable from FY 1978 to FY 1981, ranging between $63 million and $74.2 million (see Table 47). Loans increased by 24% in FY 1982, but a 25% reduction in appropriations for the overall Section 202 Pro-

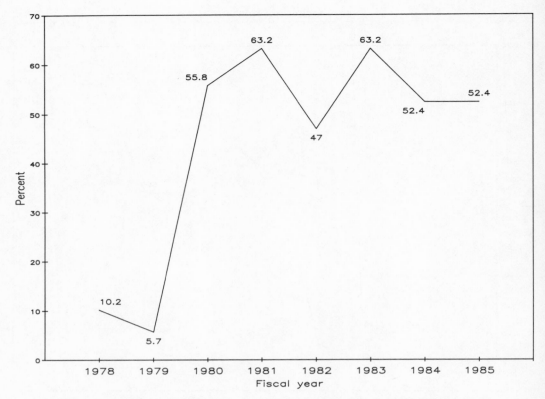

Figure 91.   Percentage of MR/DD loans of all Section 202 loans for handicapped projects: FY 1978–85.

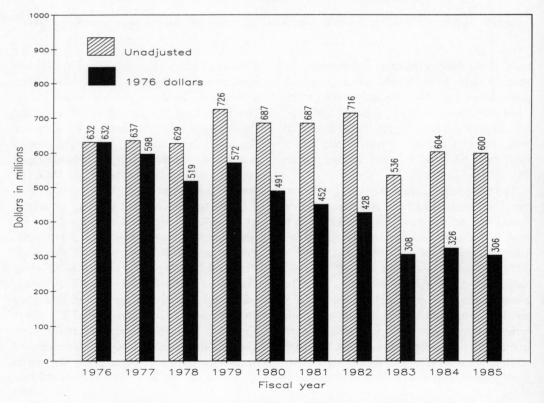

Figure 92.   Section 202 appropriations for the Elderly and Handicapped Loan Program: FY 1976–85.

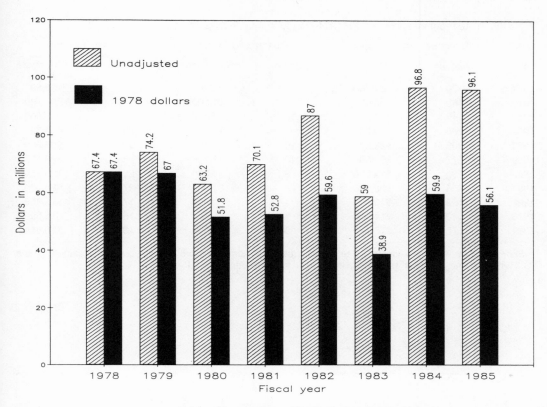

Figure 93.   Section 202 handicapped construction loans: FY 1978–85.

gram the following year was occasioned by a 32% drop in handicapped loans, the largest decline in the program's history. In FY 1984, when total Section 202 elderly and handicapped appropriations advanced by 12.7% to $604 million, handicapped loan approvals accelerated at five times that rate (64%) over the FY 1983 level. This acceleration in handicapped loans approved in FY 1984 signalled a great deal of pent-up demand after the low-water appropriations mark the previous year.

In adjusted terms, handicapped loans decreased by 23% between FY 1978 and FY 1980, rebounded by 15% by FY 1982, then plummeted almost 35% in FY 1983. The FY 1984 figure climbed 54% above the previous year's loan level. In real economic terms, the FY 1984 level, however, was actually 11% below the volume of loans approved for handicapped projects in FY 1978. Figure 93 displays the financial history of the handicapped component in the Section 202 Loan Program.

SMALL BUSINESS ACT OF 1953 AS AMENDED

In 1972, amendments to the Small Business Act, PL 92-595, authorized the Handicapped Assistance Loan (HAL) Program. Under the HAL-1 Program, direct or guaranteed loans to nonprofit organizations, including many sheltered workshops serving persons with MR/DD, were made. The HAL-2 Program provided loans to small 100% handicapped–owned businesses to construct, expand, or convert facilities; purchase building equipment or materials; and to provide working capital. In 1977, PL 95-89 authorized $100 million in federal government procurement set-asides for contracting with handicapped business concerns. Data on MR/DD participation in the HAL Programs are not available from the Small Business Administration; however, Table 48 presents data for all HAL activities funded through September 30, 1984. Since

Table 48.   HAL Program approvals: FY 1974–84 (dollars are in thousands)

FY	Direct participation loans		Guaranteed loans		Total loans	
	Number	SBA share	Number	SBA share	Number	SBA share
1974	70	$4,700	7	$800	77	$5,500
1975	69	$5,000	10	$1,100	79	$6,100
1976	140	$10,000	12	$600	152	$10,600
1977	200	$13,000	5	$1,300	205	$14,300
1978	306	$22,800	10	$1,100	316	$23,900
1979	277	$21,000	11	$1,100	288	$22,100
1980	250	$19,900	8	$300	258	$20,200
1981	254	$25,100	21	$1,800	275	$26,900
1982	168	$13,100	4	$800	172	$13,900
1983	160	$14,900	8	$1,600	168	$16,500
1984	178	$16,320	6	$544	184	$16,864

Source: Data were provided by the Small Business Administration, Handicapped Assistance Loans (C. Hertzberg and R. Lewis, personal communications, February 11, 1985).

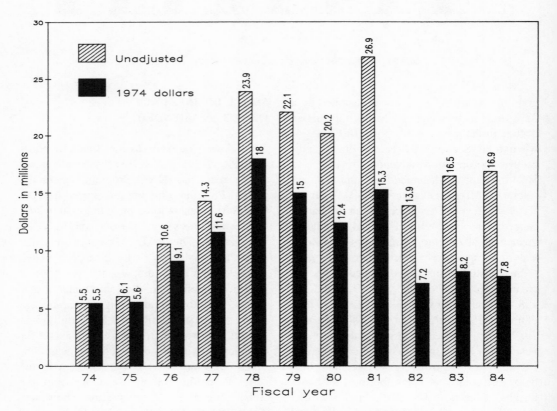

Figure 94.   Small Business Act funding for HALs: FY 1974–84.

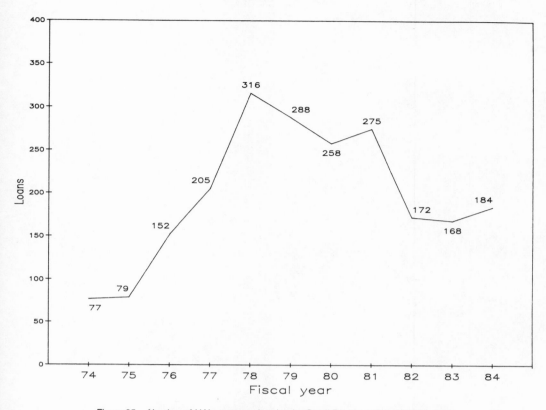

Figure 95.   Number of HALs approved under the Small Business Act: FY 1974–84.

MR/DD participation was not available, the total program data are presented for informational purposes only. (None of the HAL expenditures were included in the computations which form the basis of the author's analysis of federal government MR/DD expenditures in Chapter 9.)

The HAL Program grew from FY 1974 to FY 1978 at an average annual rate of 47% on an unadjusted basis. Total HAL loans increased from $5.5 million to $23.9 million during that period. Loan approvals peaked in FY 1981 at

$26.9 million but fell by almost 50% the following year to $13.9 million, their lowest level since FY 1976. In total, $176.9 million for 2,174 loans had been approved during the 10-year history of the program, between FY 1974 and FY 1984. In real economic terms, however, HAL loan approvals declined by 49% between FY 1981 and FY 1984 (see Figure 94).

The number of loans approved annually has ranged between 316 and 77, as depicted in Figure 95. The average individual loan approved in FY 1983 was $91,700.

Chapter 8

Information
and Coordination
Programs

THE INFORMATION/COORDINATION classification category comprises three program elements: The Secretary's Committee on Mental Retardation (SCMR); the President's Panel on Mental Retardation; and the President's Committee on Mental Retardation (PCMR). PCMR currently receives funding through the Department of Health and Human Services (DHHS) Office of Human Development Services. The President's Panel was supported for 2 years only, through $150,000 budgeted annually in FY 1962–63 by the National Institutes of Health. SCMR, and its successor, the Office of Mental Retardation Coordination (OMRC), was in continuous operation between 1963 and 1974.

It is noteworthy that as the federal MR/DD mission has grown vastly in scope and complexity since the 1960s, less funds have been expended for the support of information units and coordinative structures geared specifically toward this target population. While there are a few such mechanisms dealing with concerns of handicapped children and disabled persons in general, such as the Office of Information and Resources for the Handicapped, structures solely concerned with MR/DD issues and information have been diffused or, in the case of PCMR, slowly drained of resources. (Figure 96 graphically illustrates, in real economic terms, the federal government's declining commitment in MR/DD information and co-

ordination activities since the convening of the President's Panel.)

The Developmental Disabilities Act Amendments of 1984, Title I, Part A, Section 108 (b), however, require the DHHS secretary to establish an "interagency committee to coordinate and plan activities conducted by Federal Departments and agencies for persons with developmental disabilities." The new committee is required to meet "regularly." Membership must include representation of the Administration on Developmental Disabilities (ADD), the Office of Special Education and Rehabilitative Services, the Department of Labor, and "such other Federal Departments and agencies as the Secretary of Health and Human Services and the Secretary of Education consider appropriate." The new committee has not been given responsibility for the public dissemination of information. Funds to support the committee's activities are to be derived from ADD's salaries and expenses budget.

PRESIDENT'S PANEL
ON MENTAL RETARDATION

In October, 1961, President John F. Kennedy appointed a distinguished group of scientists, educators, physicians, lawyers, and laypersons to advise him on a program of action in mental retardation. The president asked the 27

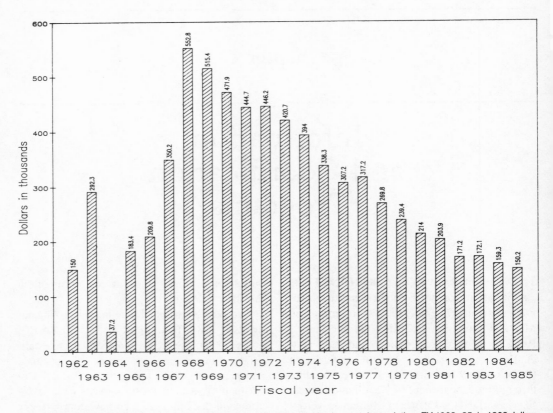

Figure 96.   Federal expenditures for information and coordination activities in mental retardation: FY 1962–85, in 1962 dollars.

appointees to report back to him before December 31, 1962.

The panel temporarily organized itself after its first meeting into two major groups: research and services. Reports were prepared over the ensuing 2 months and the panel reconvened in December, 1961. It was then decided to divide the panel's membership and focus into six task forces: prevention; education and habilitation; law and public awareness; biological research; behavioral and social research; and coordination. Public hearings were held in seven major cities and panel members visited exemplary programs throughout the United States and in Sweden, Denmark, Holland, England, and the Soviet Union. The existing body of literature on mental retardation was also reviewed as it pertained to the work of each of the six task forces.

In October, 1962, the panel issued its 200-page final report: "National Action to Combat Mental Retardation." More than 90 recommendations were presented, most of which pertained to the general mission of the Department of Health, Education, and Welfare (DHEW). Provision for strengthening HEW mental retardation programs through legislation was embodied in several of the recommendations which later became law, such as PL 88-164, the Mental Retardation Facilities and Community Mental Health Centers Construction Act of 1963.

Funds to support the panel's activities were obtained from transferring $150,000 in FY 1962 and FY 1963 from the budgets of the National Institutes of Health. The extensive degree to which the panel's recommendations ultimately became federal and state policy is impressive. The panel, for example, called for no new institutions to be constructed congregating more than 500 retarded persons.

The report ventured beyond this progressive (for the time) recommendation by insisting that retarded persons should live and be cared for in society as close to "normal community life as possible."

SECRETARY'S COMMITTEE ON MENTAL RETARDATION

The SCMR was, in part, a direct outgrowth of the *Ad Hoc* Committee on Mental Retardation, an entity established by DHEW Secretary Ovetta Hobby in early 1955 following an expression of congressional interest in mental retardation. On May 19, 1955, the committee, chaired by Joseph Douglass, who later served as executive director of the President's Committee on Mental Retardation, transmitted its report to the secretary. The committee's membership had been drawn from several DHEW operating agencies, including the Office of Education, National Institute of Neurological Diseases and Blindness, Children's Bureau, Office of Vocational Rehabilitation, National Institute of Mental Health, and Bureau of Public Assistance.

The committee issued four recommendations, the first of which was the creation of a "Departmental Committee on Mental Retardation with representation of the constituent units, with responsibility to provide the effective implementation of the Department's role . . ." in mental retardation (U.S. Department of Health, Education, and Welfare (DHEW), 1955, p. 8). The second recommendation called for the committee to be staffed within the framework of the Office of Education "so as to maintain effective intra-departmental liaison and provide exchange of information" (DHEW, 1955, p. 8). The third recommendation called for authorizing Hill-Burton Act funds to be deployed for public institutional construction projects. The fourth recommendation proposed amending Title V of the Social Security Act to increase the authorization for grants to states under the Maternal and Child Health Program. A budget of $80,000 was requested for the departmental committee, of which $3,000 was requested to

establish an *ad hoc* advisory committee to the secretary composed of agency and nonagency lay and professional representatives.

Two years later, the June 1959 "Report on Mental Retardation Programs for Fiscal Year 1960" referred to the departmental committee as having been established "early" within the Office of the Secretary (U.S. Department of Health, Education, & Welfare [DHEW], 1959, p. iii). It is not known whether all or part of the $80,000 budget request for the committee was approved for FY 1957–59, but some funds were presumably expended for committee operations.

In 1963, the departmental committee was officially reconstituted as the Secretary's Committee on Mental Retardation and served as departmental liaison to the President's Panel on Mental Retardation. The SCMR operated within the DHEW Assistant Secretary for Legislation's Office and later in the Office of the Assistant Secretary for Community and Field Services. The SCMR operated with "salaries and expenses" funds earmarked administratively in the budgets of various DHEW operating units, including the Assistant Secretary's Office.

On January 5, 1972, Elliot Richardson, then secretary of DHEW, established the Office of Mental Retardation Coordination (OMRC), which superseded the SCMR, and charged it with ministerial duties related to coordination of the department's mental retardation program. These duties explicitly included the following administrative functions:

1. Coordinating and evaluating DHEW mental retardation activities
2. Serving as a focal point for consideration of department-wide policies, programs, procedures, activities, and matters related to mental retardation
3. Serving in an advisory capacity to the secretary
4. Serving as liaison for DHEW with the President's Committee on Mental Retardation

Like its predecessor, the OMRC budget comprised funds derived from the operating bud-

Table 49.   SCMR and OMRC funding: FY 1963–74
(dollars are in thousands)

FY	SCMR	OMRC
1963	$150	
1964	$39	
1965	$198	
1966	$238	
1967	$105	
1968	$128	
1969	$120	
1970	$111	
1971	$110	
1972	$115	
1973		$115
1974		$115

Source: Data for 1963–73 are from Braddock (1973, p. 123). Data for FY 1974 is from the DHEW House appropriation hearings record on the FY 1974 budget (Office of Mental Retardation Coordination [OMRC], 1973).

gets of other DHEW agencies. (See Table 49 for SCMR and OMRC funding history.)

The tenure of OMRC was short-lived. Two years after it superseded the SCMR, it was absorbed by the statutorily created Office for Handicapped Individuals (OHI), which in turn was redesignated in 1980 as the Office of Information and Resources for the Handicapped (OIRH) and relocated to the Department of Education's Office of Special Education and Rehabilitative Services. The Rehabilitation Act of 1973, PL 93-112, had statutorily established the OHI and considerably expanded its mission, but not its budget, to address all varieties of mental and physical disability. In the process, the SCMR-OMRC coordinative and disseminative role in mental retardation had, from the secretary's vantage point and from that of concerned professionals and parents, been diffused and set adrift in the broader currents of the disability field.

PRESIDENT'S COMMITTEE
ON MENTAL RETARDATION

Established by Presidential Executive Order 11280 on May 11, 1966, the PCMR is charged with advising the president in the area of men-

tal retardation, coordinating the federal government's role in mental retardation, and developing and disseminating information on mental retardation to the general public. During 1967, its first fiscal year of operation, the PCMR budget consisted of funds drawn from budgets of the Department of Labor, Office of Economic Opportunity, and three DHEW operating agencies: The Public Health Service, Social Security Administration, and the Welfare Administration. In subsequent years, PCMR operational support has been an item in the budget of the DHEW Office of the Secretary, and it is currently administratively located within the Office of the Assistant Secretary for Human Development Services in DHEW's successor agency—the Department of Health and Human Services.

The committee consists of 21 citizen members appointed by the president for staggered 3-year terms. The secretary of DHHS serves

Table 50.   PCMR obligations history: FY 1967–85
(dollars are in thousands)

FY	Obligations
1967	$316
1968	$577
1969	$580
1970	$580
1971	$587
1972	$625
1973	$635
1974	$656
1975	$726
1976	$698
1977	$768
1978	$702
1979	$690
1980	$680
1981	$704
1982	$650
1983	$680
1984	$670
1985	$670

Source: Data for FY 1967–73 are from Braddock (1973, p. 125). Data for FY 1974–85 were provided by the PCMR (F. Krause, personal communication, October, 1983; and G. Bouthilet, personal communication, November 13, 1984).

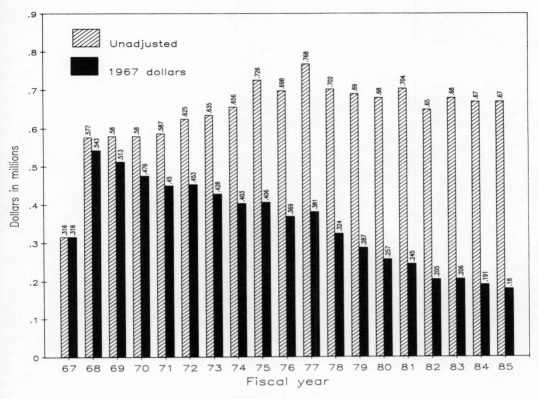

Figure 97.   PCMR budget history: FY 1967–85.

as chairman, and the following are ex-officio members: secretaries of labor and housing and urban development; attorney general; director of Action Agency; and originally, the director of the Office of Economic Opportunity (replaced by the director of the Community Services Administration, and replaced again by the secretary of education). President Richard Nixon issued a new executive order (11776) on March 28, 1974, extending the life of the committee. Executive order (12489), dated September 28, 1984, extended the committee through FY 1985.

Support for the PCMR was initiated in FY 1967. In unadjusted terms, funds obligated by the committee increased annually every year for the next decade, except in FY 1976, rising from $316,000 in FY 1967 to $768,000 in FY 1977 (see Table 50). On an adjusted basis, however, PCMR funding actually fell almost every year from FY 1968 to FY 1985. This is illustrated in Figure 97.

PART III

SUMMARY AND CONCLUSION

Chapter 9

An Analysis of Trends in Federal Spending

THE FIRST TWO chapters reviewed the history of federal financial assistance programs in mental retardation and developmental disabilities. Those chapters described the major legislative and programmatic events characterizing the evolution of federal financial policy from the early days of the Republic to the present day.

Using data presented in Chapters 3–8, this chapter summarizes global trends in federal government spending for MR/DD programs over the past 50 years. The scope of this analysis extends from the enactment of the National Industrial Recovery Act of 1933 during the first presidential term of Franklin D. Roosevelt, to the passage of FY 1985 appropriation measures at the close of President Ronald Reagan's first term.

SPENDING BY ACTIVITY CATEGORY: FY 1935–85

Figure 98 illustrates long-term trends in federal MR/DD spending for services, training, research, income maintenance, and construction activities. (Information and coordination spending is too small to be visible in Figure 98.) Data were adjusted for the impact of inflation (1950 dollars).

Services

Services program elements constituted more than half of the 53 FY 1985 elements identi-fied in the study. The services activity category included four subcomponents (FY 1985 MR/DD spending levels are indicated parenthetically): 1) vocational rehabilitation services ($134 million), primarily state grants; 2) public health services ($3.85 billion), including intermediate care facilities for the mentally retarded (ICFs/MR), noninstitutional Medicaid, Medicare, and the Civilian Health and Medical Program of the Uniformed Services; 3) human development services ($338 million), which include Developmental Disabilities Act services, Title XX social services, and volunteer services; and 4) educational services ($354 million), which include special education, vocational education, and impact aid funds.

In real economic terms, total federal funding for services increased rapidly every year between FY 1954 and 1980. In FY 1973, federal funding for services surpassed income maintenance payments for the first time. Since 1977, the margin of expenditure for services over income maintenance payments has widened every year. This has principally been due to the rapid growth of the federal ICF/MR reimbursement program. In FY 1981, the rate of MR/DD services spending growth slowed appreciably. Real growth during FY 1981–85 totaled 5.4%, or an average of 2.2% annually. This contrasted with an average rate of real economic growth from FY 1972 to FY 1980 of 15.5% per year. The reduced real growth

An adaptation of this chapter appeared in: Braddock, D. (1986c). From Roosevelt to Reagan: Federal spending for mental retardation and developmental disabilities. *American Journal of Mental Deficiency, 90*(5), 479–489.

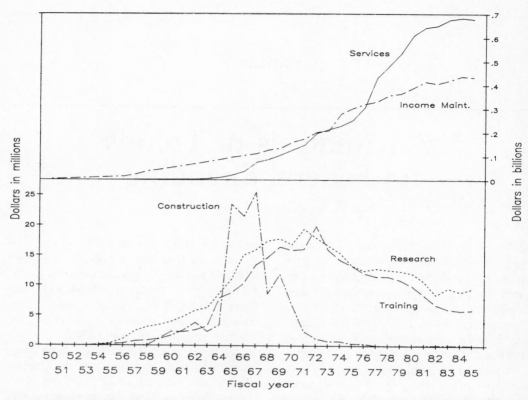

Figure 98.   Federal MR/DD spending by activity category: FY 1950–85. (In 1950 dollars). (Services and Income Maintenance are plotted against the right axis in billions of 1950 dollars; Research, Training, and Construction are plotted against the left axis in millions of 1950 dollars.)

rate since FY 1981 was primarily attributable to the diminished rate of growth in federal ICF/MR reimbursements. Federal ICF/MR payments were projected to decline slightly in real economic terms in FY 1985.

Although the overall trend in federal spending for services moved steadily upward from FY 1972 to FY 1985, this global trend concealed real economic declines in several programs during FY 1980–85 including: PL 94-142 state grants (−26%); PL 94-142 preschool incentive grants (−39%); vocational education state grants (−17%); impact aid to special education (−17%); vocational rehabilitation state grants (−.3%); DD Act state grants (−18%), and special projects (−60%); social services block grants, formerly Title XX (−37%); and Action Agency volunteer services (−15%). Total federal MR/DD spending for services in FY 1985 was $4.68

billion. This represented 60% of total MR/DD spending for all purposes in FY 1985 (see Figure 99).

Training of Personnel

The federal government has supported the training of specialists in mental retardation and developmental disabilities since FY 1954, when it began supporting the preparation of neurological specialists at the National Institute of Neurological Diseases and Blindness, now the National Institute of Neurological and Communicative Disorders and Stroke (NINCDS; U.S. House of Representatives [House], 1963). The modern training mission is divisible into four general categories of activity (FY 1985 funding levels are indicated parenthetically): 1) training of special educators ($9 million); 2) training of rehabilitation personnel ($2.6 million); 3) Na-

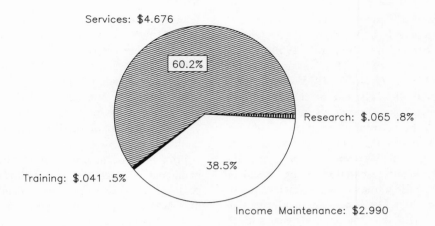

Services: $4.676

60.2%

Research: $.065 .8%

Training: $.041 .5%

38.5%

Income Maintenance: $2.990

Total: $7.773 Billion

Figure 99. Federal MR/DD spending by activity category: FY 1985. (Dollars are in billions.)

tional Institutes of Health (NIH)–sponsored training of biomedical and behavioral scientists ($3.05 million); and 4) training of University Affiliated Facility (UAF) personnel and laboratory specialists in cytogenetics ($26.1 million). The last category includes training sponsored by the Maternal and Child Health (MCH) Service in the U.S. Department of Health and Human Services (DHHS). Special education and vocational rehabilitation training is administered by the Office of Special Education and Rehabilitative Services in the U.S. Department of Education.

In real economic terms, training funds advanced every year from FY 1954 to FY 1972, except in FY 1970. After FY 1972, rehabilitation training was "decategorized" and mental retardation expenditures fell rapidly. Total training funding for FY 1985 ($40.82 million) was only one-third of the real funding level in FY 1973. Adjusted FY 1984–85 training support represented the smallest federal spending commitments in 22 years. The decline of training funds has been especially pronounced since FY 1980. In real economic terms, budget cuts were implemented in the following training programs during FY 1980–85: special education (−20%), rehabilitation (−47%), child health and human development (National Institute of Child Health and Human Development [NICHD], −25%), NINCDS

(−62%), and maternal and child health/UAF (−44%).

Research

Federal MR/DD research activity is divisible into three general categories of activity (FY 1985 funding levels are indicated parenthetically): 1) vocational rehabilitation research ($5.1 million); 2) biomedical, behavioral, and health services research ($57.2 million); and 3) educational research ($2.3 million).

Adjusted mental retardation research spending grew rapidly from FY 1954 to FY 1971. There was a 37% real dollar expansion in research funding between FY 1965 and 1966 with the establishment and funding of the NICHD, the Rehabilitation Research and Training Centers in Mental Retardation, and the special education research authority called for under Title II of PL 88-164. However, funding dropped 56% between FY 1971 and FY 1982. There were steep declines in FY 1981 (−11.5%) and FY 1982 (−20.1%). Adjusted research spending rebounded slightly in FY 1983 and FY 1985. Research retrenchment during FY 1980–85 extended to NICHD (−13%) and NINCDS (−36%). Special education research cuts totaled 70% from FY 1976 to FY 1985.

The diminution of federal funds for MR/DD

research was dramatic even in current dollar (unadjusted) terms. Funds budgeted advanced from $1.4 million in FY 1956 to $47.1 million in FY 1971. This was followed by cuts in FYs 1972, 1973, 1975, 1976, 1981, 1982, and 1984. The rate of unadjusted budget growth has slowed markedly over the years, dropping from an average of 20% annually between FY 1963 and FY 1972, to 1.1% per year between FY 1973 and FY 1982. FY 1985 research spending, based on enacted appropriations, was projected to be $64.6 million. This was an unadjusted increase of 12% over the previous year's level, primarily attributable to increased NIH funding. The president's FY 1986 budget request, however, proposed major NIH reductions in research spending (U.S. Government Printing Office, 1985).

Spending for MR/DD research as a percentage of total MR/DD expenditures has declined dramatically. From FY 1954 to FY 1972, research funds constituted between 9% and 4.5% of total federal government MR/DD expenditures. After FY 1972, federal spending for services and for income maintenance grew explosively. Research funds plunged to less than 1% of total annual MR/DD spending since FY 1981 and have remained there. Thus, as the federal government's MR/DD mission expanded, its expenditure for research relevant to that mission contracted proportionately and absolutely. In FY 1985, MR/DD research spending was .83% of total federal MR/DD spending.

Income Maintenance

Federal income maintenance programs for persons with disabilities in the United States have stemmed from five legislative achievements: 1) enactment of the Social Security Act of 1935 with its provisions for aged persons, dependent children, and blind persons contained in Titles I, IV, and X, respectively; 2) authorization in 1950 of the act's Title XIV program of Aid to the Permanently and Totally Disabled (APTD); 3) passage of the Social Security Amendments of 1956 establishing eligibility for adult disabled child (ADC) bene-

ficiaries through the disability insurance trust fund; 4) authorization of the Supplemental Security Income Program (SSI) in 1972 which extended benefits to disabled children and "federalized" administration of state-funded public assistance programs (including APTD); and 5) extension of food stamp benefits in 1976 to residents of small community living facilities.

Prior to 1950, there were no federal income maintenance programs for nonblind disabled persons. Income maintenance spending was the largest fiscal component of federal MR/DD spending during the 27-year period between FY 1950 and FY 1976—rising from $2.5 million to $1.1 billion. MR/DD payments grew another 200% over the past decade, totaling $2.99 billion in FY 1985. This represented 39% of all federal MR/DD spending (see Figure 99).

Adjusted MR/DD income maintenance spending rose every year from FY 1950 to FY 1981. The average annual real growth rate was 37% in the 1950s, 12% in the 1960s, and 10% in the 1970s. Growth decelerated during FY 1980–85 to 2.4% per year. Spending declined in real terms by 1.9% in FY 1982.

Construction

The federal government's involvement in the construction of mental retardation facilities began in 1933 with the passage of the National Industrial Recovery Act (NIRA). Enacted during the depths of the Great Depression, the law authorized grants and loans for the construction of public buildings. State mental institutions received substantial NIRA construction assistance during FY 1935–40. After the Second World War, the federal government undertook a systematic program of surplus property disposal, initially authorized by law in 1944. Numerous military installations and tuberculosis hospitals were converted into state mental retardation institutions between 1945 and 1974. Fifteen of these facilities have been closed or scheduled for closure, however (Braddock & Heller, 1985). The annual market value of surplus property transfers peaked in FY 1966–67 at $6 million and has not exceeded $1 million since FY 1975. The cumulative market value of property transfers to MR/DD use was $28.3 million over the 40-year history of the program (Office of Real Property, 1984).

The modern era of federal health care construction grants began with the Hospital Survey and Construction Act, also known as the Hill-Burton Program. Mental retardation facilities began receiving Hill-Burton assistance in FY 1958, and $32 million in federal construction grants were deployed to state institutions and nonprofit community facilities between FY 1958 and FY 1971 (U.S. Department of Health, Education, and Welfare, 1972). In 1963, Congress enacted the Mental Retardation Facilities and Community Mental Health Centers Construction Act (PL 88-164). Title I of the act was the first federal legislation dedicated exclusively to the construction of mental health and mental retardation facilities. Over the next decade, $155.8 million in federal funds were obligated for the construction of mental retardation research centers ($27 million), UAFs ($38.6 million), and community facilities ($90.2 million). An additional $5.1 million in construction funding were expended during FY 1972–76 under provisions of the Developmental Disabilities Services and Facilities Construction Act of 1970 (PL 91-517).

Federal construction spending peaked in FY 1967 at $47.3 million and declined rapidly thereafter. Federal reimbursements under the $2.66 billion ICF/MR Program, however, were discussed in the services activity category of this analysis. The cost component of ICF/MR reimbursements attributable to construction amortization is significant but unknown. Gettings and Mitchell (1980) identified cumulative state-federal mental retardation construction spending of nearly $1 billion between FY 1977 and FY 1979, most of which was attributable to ICF/MR–related activity.

Information and Coordination

The information-coordination activity category comprises three program elements: The Secretary's Committee on Mental Retardation (SCMR); the President's Panel on Mental Retardation; and the President's Committee on Mental Retardation (PCMR). The President's Panel was supported for 2 years only, from $150,000 budgeted annually in FY 1962–63 in the budget of the NIH. The SCMR, and its successor, the Office of Mental Retardation Coordination (OMRC), was in continuous operation between FY 1963 and FY 1974. SCMR-OMRC funding averaged $130,000 annually. The unit was superseded in FY 1974 by the Office for Handicapped Individuals (OHI), which was then terminated a decade later.

Support for the PCMR was initiated in FY 1967. In unadjusted terms, committee funding increased steadily from FY 1967 to FY 1977—rising from $316,000 to $768,000. On an adjusted basis, PCMR funding fell every year from FY 1968 to FY 1985, declining 67% over the 17-year period. PCMR's budget fell another 30% in real terms during FY 1980–85. Its budget was $670,000 in FY 1985. As the federal mission in MR/DD grew in scope and complexity over time, less emphasis was placed on centralized informational and coordinative structures, as was the case with research and training activities.

MEASURING FEDERAL MR/DD FISCAL EFFORT

MR/DD Percentage of the Total Federal Budget

The percentage of the federal government's total annual budget devoted to financing MR/DD activities, except for a momentary hesitation in FY 1975, advanced every year from FY 1950 to FY 1981 (see top line of Figure 100). The annual rate of the advance averaged 30% per year during FY 1950–56; 23% during FY 1956–67; and 8% during FY 1967–81. MR/DD spending growth more than tripled between FY 1967 and FY 1981 as a percentage of total federal spending, and there were very large absolute gains in total MR/DD spending.

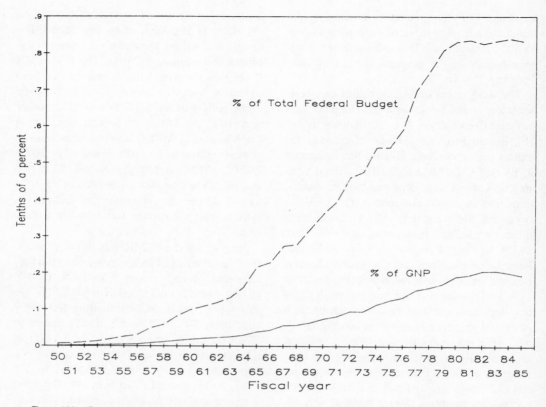

Figure 100.   Percentages of the total federal budget and of the GNP expended for MR/DD activities: FY 1950–85.

In FY 1982, however, the MR/DD share of total federal disbursements fell detectably for the first time, by 1%—to .83% of total federal expenditures. The MR/DD share of federal spending remained at that level in FY 1983, advanced marginally to .84% in FY 1984, and was projected to revert to the FY 1983 level in FY 1985. Although MR/DD spending as a percentage of the total federal budget was basically flat during FY 1981–85, MR/DD spending increased 6.2% as a percentage of overall federal domestic spending (i.e., from 1.0739% in FY 1981 to 1.1405% in FY 1985).

MR/DD Share of the GNP

As a percentage of the gross national product (GNP), mental retardation and developmental disabilities expenditures advanced at an average annual rate of 35% during FY 1950–56 (see bottom line of Figure 100). Between FY

1956 and FY 1967, the rate of growth slowed to 25% per annum; and during FY 1967–81 it dropped to 9% per year. In FY 1973, it fell marginally but quickly resumed its upward momentum from FY 1974 to FY 1981.

In FY 1982 and FY 1983, however, the MR/DD share peaked at .21% of the GNP. Then, it declined the next 2 years. During FY 1982–84 total federal MR/DD expenditures were flat in real economic terms but the nation's total economic output (or GNP) climbed 8%. In the course of its strong recovery from the 1981 recession, the U.S. economy expanded appreciably faster than did federal MR/DD expenditures. This had not occurred in the previous 30 years.

SUMMARY OF FY 1985 MR/DD SPENDING

Federal spending for mental retardation and developmental disabilities in FY 1985 was

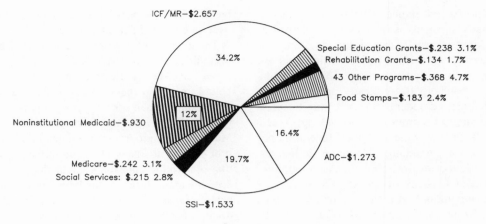

ICF/MR—$2.657

34.2%

Special Education Grants—$.238 3.1%
Rehabilitation Grants—$.134 1.7%

43 Other Programs—$.368 4.7%

Food Stamps—$.183 2.4%

12%

16.4%

Noninstitutional Medicaid—$.930

19.7%

ADC—$1.273

Medicare—$.242 3.1%
Social Services: $.215 2.8%

SSI—$1.533

Total: $7.773 Billion

Figure 101.   Federal MR/DD spending by program: FY 1985. (Dollars are in billions.)

$7.773 billion. This was half of total public (federal-state-local) expenditures for MR/DD in the United States (Braddock & Hemp, 1986). The FY 1985 MR/DD spending figure consisted of $6.499 billion in congressionally appropriated funds and $1.274 billion in Social Security trust funds. The Department of Health and Human Services and the Department of Education were responsible for administering 97% of all federal mental retardation and developmental disabilities expenditures in FY 1985.

The largest federal MR/DD program in FY 1985, accounting for over one-third of all federal MR/DD spending, was the ICF/MR Program, with total projected reimbursements of $2.657 billion. Three-fourths of all federal ICF/MR funding in FY 1985 provided support for clients placed in state-operated institutions (Braddock, Hemp, & Howes, 1985). Another one-third of total federal MR/DD spending consisted of the total of SSI payments and ADC benefits. Six other programs collectively accounted for one-fourth of total MR/DD funds budgeted in FY 1985: noninstitutional Medicaid, Medicare, PL 94-142 state grants, social services, food stamps, and rehabilitation state grants. Nine programs thus accounted for 95% of all federal MR/DD spending in FY 1985. This is illustrated in Figure 101.

CONCLUSION

The federal government has supported MR/DD activities for more than half a century, but the majority of the cumulative total of $62 billion budgeted for this purpose in unadjusted terms has been expended since FY 1981. Even in real economic terms, 53% of all federal MR/DD funds expended have been deployed since FY 1979. These remarkable statistics are the product of the prodigious expansion in federal MR/DD spending for services and income maintenance from FY 1974 to 1981.

The "Institutional Bias" of Federal Financial Assistance

The extensive degree to which contemporary federal spending for services consists of funds expended for care in state-operated institutions is an important finding. In FY 1985, 41% of the $4.68 billion in federal spending for MR/DD services supported approximately 100,000 placements in public institutions nationwide. The remaining federal funds (59%) helped finance services for the vastly larger population of individuals with mental retardation residing in noninstitutional settings. There are, for example, 630,000 noninstitutionalized mentally retarded recipients of Supplemental Security Income alone.

The federal emphasis on financing institutional placements is only partly explained by the excess cost of caring for the somewhat greater severity of the typical institutional resident's disability versus that of his noninstitutional counterpart. A clearly articulated and well-financed federal policy commitment to community integration is also lacking. Absent the likelihood of much "new" federal money to finance community integration initiatives, some advocates, including the Association for Retarded Citizens of the United States, are focusing political attention on the institutional bias in the disbursement of federal ICF/MR funds. FY 1985 federal ICF/MR reimbursements are projected at $2.657 billion—three-fourths of these funds support institutional placements. In today's restrained budgetary environment, the appeal to advocates of diverting a substantial share of existing ICF/MR institutional reimbursements to community care objectives is self-evident. This appeal recently manifested itself in the introduction of the Community and Family Living Amendments of 1985 in the U.S. Congress (S.873 and H.R.2902). Various organized interests have also suggested alternatives for financing additional community services by expanding the scope and flexibility of the Medicaid Home and Community-Based Waiver Program (Censoni, 1985; Turnbull, 1985).

End of an Era

Money, of course, is only one indicator of the federal government's performance over time, and of federal concern for persons with MR/DD. Merely because more funds are deployed to community settings does not ensure superior client outcomes. But during the early stages of the nationwide movement to implement community-based services in the United States, the record of public expenditure is the best single indicator of the political progress being made. This book has demonstrated that that progress has, at least temporarily, plateaued. Whether or not this plateau presages a long-term future trend cannot be predicted accurately; but this should be the subject of a continuing scholarly effort to carefully monitor

public MR/DD spending in the United States over an extended period of time.

The interests of persons with developmental disabilities are, to paraphrase the President's Panel on Mental Retardation, inextricably bound up within the scores of health, educational, and human services programs presently administered by the federal government. Many of these programs originated in the spirit of Roosevelt's New Deal and in the legislation of Lyndon Johnson's Great Society. Indeed the major thrust of the lobbying effort on behalf of persons with MR/DD over the past 2 decades has been to press for favorable legislative and regulatory provisions incorporated into Great Society enactments.

The diffusion of legislative provisions and administrative directives favorable to MR/DD interests has been extensive at the federal level. The scale and scope of the 82 relevant federal programs identified in this book are testimony to the general responsiveness of our political institutions, to the effectiveness of professional and consumer organizations, and to the underlying humanism uniting the MR/DD field. Only a generation ago, there was no federal funding for MR/DD programs; now there is substantial support for services and income maintenance. This is the long view—looking at the trends over the 50-year era from Roosevelt to Reagan.

The short-term view is another matter. The diffusion of federal MR/DD programs across the broad panorama of governmental operations—from health care to housing loans—has brought with it new vulnerabilities. There is now a great deal that can be taken away; and, there are great expectations for community integration on the part of both professionals and consumers. The FY 1981–85 period has been sobering to a field that has experienced essentially uninterrupted real economic growth in federal spending for the quarter-century between FY 1955 and FY 1980. Since FY 1981, significantly more federal resources have been allocated to underwrite national defense; and less funds have been deployed for domestic activities generally, including MR/DD programs. In relation to overall domestic budget trends since FY 1981, total federal MR/DD spending has been relatively strong. The primary reason for the field's overall fiscal strength is the entitlement features of the SSI/ADC and Medicaid programs.

Research Renewal

It is stressed, however, that discretionary federal support for MR/DD research and training activities has been steadily declining in real economic terms for nearly 15 years. To describe this long-term decline as a crisis is an understatement; to attribute its cause solely to the present administration or even to the recent deep recession is factually incorrect. Four consecutive presidential administrations (of both political parties), dating back to Richard M. Nixon and budgetary decisions implemented during his first presidential term, have presided over the demise of MR/DD research and personnel training as priorities of the federal government. In recent years, MR/DD research and training activities have been fiscally deemphasized along with scientific research and training in general. The movement toward noncategorical research and training support in special education and vocational rehabilitation, like the general move toward block grants for financing services, has also contributed to diminished federal funding of MR/DD research and training activities.

The success of this nation's efforts to prevent mental retardation and other developmental disabilities and to provide humane, professional care in integrated community settings is dependent on the adoption of long-term federal financial incentives, on the systematic expansion and application of the field's knowledge-base, and on an adequate and continuing supply of caring and competent personnel. Thus, it is essential for MR/DD research and training activities to be re-established as funding priorities of the U.S. government. Achieving this objective will require MR/DD researchers to join with those in the general social and biomedical sciences to press for increased support for research and training in general. Equally important, achieving this objective will also require the MR/DD research community to more clearly and convincingly articulate why scientific research and training is an efficacious investment of scarce public resources.

Epilogue

WHAT A MAGNIFICENT job David Braddock has done in compressing in clear outline an avalanche of data on programs and expenditures whose magnitude truly surpasses understanding. As I proceeded through his many tables and figures, time and time again I stopped to think "What would John E. Fogarty have thought about these vast expenditures?" John E. Fogarty, the bricklayer and union steward, who, as chairman of the House Appropriations Subcommittee on Labor and Health, Education, and Welfare, became one of the nation's leading strategists in human services in the 1950s and a powerful, albeit conservative, advocate for persons with mental retardation and their families. Fogarty cared deeply about people, but also assumed for himself and demanded from others a diligent stewardship and accountability toward expenditure of public funds; his million dollar appropriations were scrutinized meticulously by him as they were expended. By contrast, in the 1980s, the Title XIX ICF/MR machine spewed out billions of tax dollars with little regard to their utilization by the states.

Writing in the concluding chapter of the first edition of *Changing Patterns in Residential Services for the Mentally Retarded* (Kugel & Wolfensberger, 1969), I said, "the Government . . . can give new directions by exercising greater discrimination in its granting practices. Federal legislation is needed which not merely encourages new service patterns but discourages continuation of the old ones. . . . Those states could be given priority which are actively supporting dispersal and integration of residential services, rather than states which continue to enlarge existing large institutions or which place new residential facilities in remote locations." Yet today, masses of Title XIX federal funds encourage the state of New York to enlarge its institutions by building so-called community residences right on the grounds of existing oversized institutions now posing as developmental centers, and some other states are following suit.

Now that the new drive for federal deficit reduction, fortified by the Gramm-Rudman-Hollings Act, is requiring a re-thinking of budgetary priorities, David Braddock confronts us most helpfully with a frightening picture of a lopsided expenditure pattern that, for the past several years, seems to have lost its sense of direction. But in considering what the future should bring to persons with mental retardation and their families, we should reject the supposition that what is past is prologue and instead hold with Edmund Burke that you cannot plan for the future by the past. We need to shift gears and priorities and focus less on accommodating the residential establishment, be it public or private, and more on enabling the persons in residences to fulfill their individual potentials, instead of subjecting them to a repressive, regulatory system that was really not drawn up in their interest. We need to rediscover the family and its strength, resourcefulness, and caring (Dybwad, 1982), and build up a cost-effective system of support.

Above all, we need to recognize a new source of strength—the self-advocacy movement, as represented by groups such as People First, United Together, or Speaking for Ourselves. The Oettinger Foundation was in the forefront of sensitive thinking in this area when, as early as 1973, it provided a grant to make possible meetings of a statewide group of self-advocates. The grant was microscopic compared to federal levels of disbursements, but its cost-effectiveness was exceedingly high, leading to sustained advocacy action.

As is the case in other areas of the disability field, patients and clients have become persons, far more aware of their problems than was ever believed possible, far more able to look after themselves than was ever thought possible. Thus, their voices must be heard if future years are to bring us more appropriate, more cost-effective, and more person-related programs, whatever the sources of funding.

Gunnar Dybwad, Ph.D.
Professor Emeritus of Human Development
Heller School
Brandeis University

References

Bibliographical Citations

Abeson, A., Bolick, N., & Haas, J. (1975). *A primer on due process*. Reston, VA: Council for Exceptional Children.

Advisory Commission on Intergovernmental Relations. (1984). *Significant features of fiscal federalism* (1982–83 ed.). Washington, DC: Author.

American Bar Association. (1978). Introduction. In *Collection of data on public expenditures for care of the mentally disabled* (pp. 1–3). Chicago: Division of Public Service Activities.

Boggs, E.M. (1971). Federal legislation. In J. Wortis (Ed.), *Mental retardation: III* (pp. 103–127). New York: Grune & Stratton.

Boggs, E.M. (1972). Federal legislation (Conclusion). In J. Wortis (Ed.), *Mental retardation: IV* (pp. 165–206). New York: Grune & Stratton.

Braddock, D. (1973). Mental retardation funds: An analysis of federal policy. Unpublished doctoral dissertation, University of Texas at Austin, Department of Special Education.

Braddock, D. (1974). Mental retardation funds: An analysis of federal policy. In J. Wortis (Ed.), *Mental retardation and developmental disabilities: An annual review* (Vol. 6, pp. 106–146). New York: Brunner/Mazel.

Braddock, D. (1977). *Opening closed doors*. Reston, VA: Council for Exceptional Children.

Braddock, D. (1981). Deinstitutionalization of the mentally retarded: Trends in public policy. *Hospital and Community Psychiatry, 32*(9), 607–615.

Braddock, D. (1986a). Federal assistance for mental retardation and developmental disabilities through 1961. *Mental Retardation, 24*(3), 175–182.

Braddock, D. (1986b). Federal assistance for mental retardation and developmental disabilities: The modern era, 1962–84. *Mental Retardation, 24*(4).

Braddock, D. (1986c). From Roosevelt to Reagan: Federal spending for mental retardation and developmental disabilities. *American Journal of Mental Deficiency, 90*(5), 479–489.

Braddock, D. (1986d). The transformation of governmental spending patterns. In R. Kugel (Ed.), *Changing patterns in residential services to persons with mental retardation*. Washington, DC: President's Committee on Mental Retardation.

Braddock, D., & Fujiura, G. (in press). State financial effort for mental retardation institutional and community services. *American Journal of Mental Deficiency*.

Braddock, D., & Heller, T. (1985). The closure of mental retardation institutions. Part I: Trends in the United States. *Mental Retardation, 23*(4), 168–176.

Braddock, D., & Hemp, R. (1986). Intergovernmental spending for mental retardation and developmental disabilities in the United States: Results of a nationwide study. *Hospital and Community Psychiatry, 37*(7), 702–707.

Braddock, D., Hemp, R., & Howes, R. (1984). *Public expenditures for mental retardation and developmental disabilities in the United States: State profiles*. Chicago: University of Illinois at Chicago, Institute for the Study of Developmental Disabilities, Evaluation and Public Policy Analysis Program.

Braddock, D., Hemp, R., & Howes, R. (1985). *Public expenditures for mental retardation and developmental disabilities in the United States: Analytic summary*. Chicago: University of Illinois at Chicago, Institute for the Study of Developmental Disabilities, Evaluation and Public Policy Analysis Program.

Braddock, D., Hemp, R., & Howes, R. (1986). Direct costs of institutional care in the United States. *Mental Retardation, 24*(1), 9–17.

Braddock, D., Hemp, R., & Howes, R. (in press). Financing community services in the United States: Results of a nationwide study. *Mental Retardation*.

Bureau of Economic Analysis. (1981, July). *National income and product accounts*. Washington, DC: U.S. Department of Commerce.

Bureau of Economic Analysis. (1983, July). *Survey of current business*. Washington, DC: U.S. Department of Commerce, Bureau of Economic Analysis.

Bureau of Economic Analysis. (1984, April). *Survey of current business*. Washington, DC: U.S. Department of Commerce.

Caiden, N. (1976). *Collection of data on public expenditure for care of the mentally disabled*.

Memorandum prepared for Commission on the Mentally Disabled, American Bar Association, Division of Public Service Activities, Washington, DC.

Castellani, P. (in press). *Political economy of developmental disabilities.* Baltimore: Paul H. Brookes Publishing Co.

Censoni, B. (1985). *Statement of testimony on the deficit reduction amendments of 1985 on behalf of the National Association of State Mental Retardation Program Directors.* Alexandria, VA: The National Association of State Mental Retardation Program Directors.

Conley, R.W., & Noble, J.H. (1985, April 9–10). *Severely handicapped Americans: Victims of misguided policies.* Paper presented at the Economics of Disability Meeting, U.S. Department of Education, Office of the Assistant Secretary for Special Education and Rehabilitation Services, National Institute of Handicapped Research, Washington, DC.

Consortium for Citizens with Developmental Disabilities. (1984). *Analysis of the president's FY 1985 budget proposals.* Washington, DC: Consortium Task Force on Budget and Appropriations.

Dybwad, G. (1969). Action implications in the U.S.A. today. In R. Kugel & W. Wolfensberger (Eds.), *Changing patterns in residential services for the mentally retarded* (pp. 383–428). Washington, DC: President's Committee on Mental Retardation.

Dybwad, G. (1982). The rediscovery of the family. *Mental Retardation* (Canada), *32*(1), 19–30.

Easton, D. (1965). *A framework for political analysis.* Englewood Cliffs, NJ: Prentice-Hall.

Falk, I.S., & Geddes, A.E. (1941). Medical care in public welfare programs. *Medical Care, 1*(1), 64–77.

Gettings, R. (1981). *Federal funding inquiry: Congressional action on the Reagan budget proposals.* Arlington, VA: National Association of State Mental Retardation Program Directors.

Gettings, R., & Mitchell, D. (1980). *Trends in capital expenditures for mental retardation facilities.* Arlington, VA: National Association of State Mental Retardation Program Directors.

Gilhool, T. (1976). The uses of courts and of lawyers. In R. Kugel & A. Shearer (Eds.), *Changing patterns in residential services for the mentally retarded* (2nd edition, pp. 155–184). Washington, DC: President's Committee on Mental Retardation.

Gray, V. (1980). The determinants of public policy: A reappraisal of the literature. In T. Dye & V. Gray (Eds.), *The determinants of public policy* (pp. 215–222). Lexington, MA: Lexington Books.

Head Start Bureau (1982). *The status of handicapped children in Head Start programs—eighth annual report to Congress* (Publication No. 12). Washington, DC: Department of Health and Human Services, Office of Human Development Services, Administration on Children, Youth, and Families.

Heal, L., & Fujiura, G. (1984). Methodological considerations in research on residential alternatives for developmentally disabled persons. In N.R. Ellis & N.W. Bray (Eds.), *International review of research in mental retardation.* Orlando, FL: Academic Press.

Herr, S. (1983). *Rights and advocacy for retarded people.* Lexington, MA: D.C. Heath.

Herr, S. (1984). *Issues in human rights.* New York: Young Adult Institute Press.

Herr, S., Arons, R., & Wallace, R. (1983). *Legal rights and mental health care.* Lexington, MA: D.C. Heath.

Hofferbert, R. (1972). State and community policy studies: A review of comparative input-output analysis. In J.A. Robinson (Ed.), *Political Science Annual* (Vol. 3, pp. 3–72). Indianapolis: Bobbs-Merrill.

Hornmuth, R.P. (1964). Community clinics for the mentally retarded. In U.S. Children's Bureau (Ed.), *Historical perspective on mental retardation during the decade 1954–64* (pp. 49–53). Washington, DC: U.S. Children's Bureau.

Johnson, R. (1975). Research objectives for policy analysis. In K. Dolbeare (Ed.), *Public policy evaluation* (pp. 75–94). Beverly Hills: Sage Publications.

Kakalik, J.S., Furry, W.S., Thomas, M.A., & Carney, M.F. (1981). *The costs of special education: Summary of study findings.* Santa Monica, CA: The Rand Corporation.

Lakin, K.C. (1979). *Demographic studies of residential facilities for the mentally retarded: An historical review of methodologies and findings.* Minneapolis: University of Minnesota, Department of Educational Psychology.

LaVor, M. (1975). Federal legislation for exceptional persons: A history. In F. Weintraub, A. Abeson, J. Ballard, & M. LaVor (Eds.), *Public policy and the education of exceptional children* (pp. 96–111). Reston, VA: Council for Exceptional Children.

Lesser, A. (1964). Health services—accomplishments and outlook. In U.S. Children's Bureau (Ed.), *Historical perspective on mental retardation* (Publication No. 426-1964, pp. 176–182). Washington, DC: U.S. Children's Bureau.

Litvin, M., & Browning, P. (1977). *Public assistance and mental retardation through 1976.* Eugene, OR: Rehabilitation Research and Training Center.

Lundberg, E.O. (1917). *A social study of mental defectives in New Castle County, Delaware* (Publication No. 24). Washington, DC: Children's Bureau.

Mackie, R. (1969). *Special education in the United States: Statistics: 1948–66*. New York: Teachers College Press.

Martin, E.W. (1968). Breakthrough for the handicapped: Legislative history. *Exceptional Children, 34*(7), 493–503.

Masland, R., Sarason, S., & Gladwin, T. (1958). *Mental subnormality*. New York: Basic Books.

Mountin, J.W. (1949). The history and functions of the United States Public Health Service. In J.S. Simmons (Ed.), *Public health in the world today* (pp. 83–92). Cambridge, MA: Harvard University Press.

Mugge, R. (1964). The people who receive APTD. *Welfare in Review, 2*(11), 1–14.

Nathan, R., & Doolittle, F. (1984). Overview: Effects of the Reagan domestic program on states and localities. Princeton, NJ: Princeton University, Urban and Regional Research Center.

National Association of State Mental Retardation Program Directors. (1984). Congress approves disability reforms. *Capitol Capsule, 14*(9), 1–3.

National Association of State Mental Retardation Program Directors. (1985, April 17). *Federal funding inquiry: Federal constraints on state Medicaid outlays for MR/DD recipients*. Alexandria, VA: Author.

Office for Handicapped Individuals. (1975). *Mental retardation programs: Department of Health, Education, and Welfare supplementary data for FY 1976 house appropriations subcommittee hearings*. Washington, DC: Author.

Office for Handicapped Individuals. (1976). *Mental retardation programs: Department of Health, Education, and Welfare supplementary data for FY 1977 house appropriations subcommittee hearings*. Washington, DC: Author.

Office for Handicapped Individuals. (1977). *Mental retardation programs: Department of Health, Education, and Welfare supplementary data for FY 1978 house appropriations subcommittee hearings*. Washington, DC: Author.

Office for Handicapped Individuals. (1980). *Summary of existing legislation relating to the handicapped* (Publication No. E-80-22014). Washington, DC: U.S. Department of Education.

Office of Child Development, Research and Evaluation Division. (1972). *Head Start 1969–1970: A descriptive report of programs and participants* (pp. 97–98). Washington, DC: Department of Health, Education and Welfare, Research and Evaluation Division, Office of Child Development.

Office of Mental Retardation Coordination. (1972).

Mental retardation sourcebook (Publication No. 05, pp. 73–81). Washington, DC: Department of Health, Education, and Welfare.

Office of Mental Retardation Coordination. (1973). *Mental retardation programs: Department of Health, Education, and Welfare supplementary data for FY 1974 house appropriations subcommittee hearings*. Washington, DC: Author.

Office of Mental Retardation Coordination. (1974). *Mental retardation programs: Department of Health, Education, and Welfare supplementary data for FY 1975 house appropriations subcommittee hearings*. Washington, DC: Author.

Office of Real Property. (1984). Administrative records on mental retardation surplus property transfers. Washington, DC: Department of Health and Human Services.

Pennsylvania Association for Retarded Children v. Commonwealth of Pennsylvania, 343 F. Supp. 279 (1972).

President's Panel on Mental Retardation. (1962). *National action to combat mental retardation*. Washington, DC: U.S. Government Printing Office.

President's Task Force on the Mentally Handicapped. (1970). *Action against mental disability*. Washington, DC: U.S. Government Printing Office.

Rose, D. (1973). National and local forces in state politics: The implications of multi-level policy analysis. *The American Political Science Review, 68*(4), 1162–1173.

Secretary's Committee on Mental Retardation. (1963). *Mental retardation activities of the Department of Health, Education, and Welfare*. Washington, DC: U.S. Government Printing Office.

Secretary's Committee on Mental Retardation. (1965). *Mental retardation activities of the Department of Health, Education, and Welfare*. Washington, DC: U.S. Government Printing Office.

Secretary's Committee on Mental Retardation. (1971). *Mental retardation activities of the U.S. Department of Health, Education and Welfare: 1970*. Washington, DC: Author.

Short, C.W., & Stanley-Brown, R. (1939). *A summary of the architecture of projects constructed by federal and other governmental bodies between 1933 and 1939 with the assistance of the Public Works Administration*. Washington, DC: U.S. Government Printing Office.

Social Security Administration. (1981). *Social security bulletin, annual statistical supplement, 1981* (Publication No. 13-117). Washington, DC: U.S. Government Printing Office.

Social Security Administration. (1983). *Social security bulletin annual statistical supplement,*

1983 (Publication No. 13-117). Washington, DC: U.S. Government Printing Office.

Social Security Board. (1946). *Recommendations of the Children's Bureau Advisory Committee on services to crippled children, December, 1935 to April, 1946.* Washington, DC: Author.

Stedman, D. (1976). State councils on developmental disabilities. *Exceptional Children, 42*(4), 186–192.

Stedman, D., Richmond, J., & Tarjan, G. (1984). *Minutes of the annual meeting of the National Advisory Committee of the Illinois Institute for Developmental Disabilities.* Chicago: Office of the Director of the Illinois Institute for Developmental Disabilities.

Surveys and Research Corporation. (1965). *Mental retardation program statistics of the U.S. Department of Health, Education, and Welfare in 1964.* Washington DC: Author.

Treadway, W.L., & Lundberg, E.O. (1919). *Mental defect in a rural county* (Publication No. 48). Washington, DC: Children's Bureau.

Trudeau, E. (1971). *Digest of state and federal laws: Education of handicapped children.* Reston, VA: Council for Exceptional Children.

Turnbull, H.R. (1985). *Statement of testimony at a hearing on budget reconciliation before the U.S. Senate Finance Committee on behalf of the Consortium Concerned with Developmental Disabilities.* Washington, DC: Consortium Concerned with Developmental Disabilities.

U.S. Children's Bureau. (1915). *Mental defectives in the District of Columbia* (Publication No. 13). Washington, DC: Author.

U.S. Children's Bureau. (1963). *Children, problems, and services in the child welfare programs* (Publication No. 403-1963). Washington, DC: Author.

U.S. Children's Bureau. (1964). A history of Children's Bureau activities in behalf of mentally retarded children. In *Historical perspective on mental retardation during the decade 1954–64* (Publication No. 426–1964, pp. 1–11). Washington, DC: Author.

U.S. Children's Bureau. (1981). *National study of social services to handicapped children and their families.* Washington, DC: Author.

U.S. Department of Education. (1982). *Secretary's report on vocational education.* Washington, DC: Author.

U.S. Department of Health, Education, & Welfare. (1955). *Report of the ad hoc committee on mental retardation on proposed programs, activities, services, and budget estimates in the field of mental retardation—Fiscal Year 1957.* Washington, DC: DHEW, Office of the Secretary, Office of Program Analysis.

U.S. Department of Health, Education, and Welfare. (1959). *Mental retardation programs and services of the U.S. Department of Health, Education, and Welfare: FY 1960.* Washington, DC: Author, Office of Program Analysis.

U.S. Department of Health, Education, & Welfare. (1972). *Willowbrook report.* Washington, DC: Author.

U.S. Department of Health, Education, & Welfare, Health Services and Mental Health Administration. (1972). *Hill-Burton project register.* Washington, DC: DHEW, Health Care Facilities Service, Office of Program Planning and Analysis.

U.S. Department of Health and Human Services. (1946). *Recommendations of the Children's Bureau Advisory Committee on services to crippled children. December, 1935, to April, 1946.* Washington, DC: Author.

U.S. Department of Health and Human Services. (1981). *Social Security bulletin, annual statistical supplement.* Washington, DC: U.S. Government Printing Office.

U.S. Department of Health and Human Services. (1983). *Social Security bulletin, annual statistical supplement* (SSA Publication No. 13-11700). Washington, DC: U.S. Government Printing Office.

U.S. General Accounting Office. (1982). *Early observations on block grant implementation.* Gaithersberg, MD: General Accounting Office, Document Handling and Information Services Facility.

U.S. Government Printing Office. (1985). *The budget of the United States government: 1985.* Washington, DC: Author.

U.S. House of Representatives, Committee on Ways and Means, Social Security Technical Staff. (1946). *Issues in social security.* Washington, DC: U.S. Government Printing Office.

U.S. House of Representatives; Committee on Appropriations; Subcommittee on Appropriations for the Departments of Labor, and Health, Education, and Welfare. (1955). *Hearings on FY 1956 appropriations: Part one.* Washington, DC: U.S. Government Printing Office.

U.S. House of Representatives; Committee on Appropriations; Subcommittee on Labor, and Health, Education and Welfare. (1963). *Supplemental appropriations to combat mental retardation.* Washington, DC: U.S. Government Printing Office.

U.S. House of Representatives, Ad Hoc House Subcommittee on Handicapped Children. (1966). *Hearings.* Washington, DC: U.S. Government Printing Office.

U.S. House of Representatives. (1978). *Committee on appropriations (FY 1979), on the Depart-*

ments of Labor and Health, Education, and Welfare: Part 2. Washington, DC: U.S. Government Printing Office.

U.S. House of Representatives. (1979). *Committee on appropriations (FY 1980), subcommittee on the Departments of Labor, Health, Education and Welfare: Part 2.* Washington, DC: U.S. Government Printing Office.

U.S. House of Representatives; Committee on Appropriations (FY 1981); Department of Health, Education, and Welfare Appropriations Subcommittee, *Hearings.* (1980). Washington, DC: U.S. Government Printing Office.

U.S. House of Representatives. (1981). *Committee on appropriations (FY 1982), subcommittee on the Departments of Labor, Health, Education and Welfare: Part 2.* Washington, DC: U.S. Government Printing Office.

U.S. House of Representatives. (1982). *Committee on appropriations (FY 1983), subcommittee on the Departments of Labor, Health, Education and Welfare: Part 2.* Washington, DC: U.S. Government Printing Office.

U.S. House of Representatives, Committee on Appropriations (FY 1984), Department of Health & Human Services Appropriations Subcommittee. (1983). *Hearings.* Washington, DC: U.S. Government Printing Office.

U.S. House of Representatives. (1984). *Conference report on the Developmental Disabilities Act of 1984.* Washington, DC: U.S. Government Printing Office.

White House. (1971, November 16). *Statement on mental retardation of President Richard M. Nixon.* Washington, DC: White House Press Office.

White House Conference on Handicapped Individuals. (1980). *Final report.* Washington, DC: Office for Handicapped Individuals.

Wieck, C., & Bruininks, R. (1980). *The cost of public and community residential care for mentally retarded people in the United States.* Minneapolis: University of Minnesota, Department of Psychoeducational Studies, Developmental Disabilities Project on Residential Services and Community Adjustment.

Wildavsky, A. (1975). *The politics of the budgetary process* (rev. ed.). Boston: Little, Brown.

Wyatt v. Stickney, 344 F. Supp 387, 395 (M.D. Ala. 1972), *aff'd sub* nom. Wyatt v Aderholt, 503 F.2d 1305 (5th cir. 1974).

Federal Agency Respondents

*Advisory Commission
on Intergovernmental Relations*

Michael W. Lawson, Taxation and Finance Unit

Congressional Budget Office

George Arnold, Budget Analysis Division, Scorekeeping Unit, chief of

Small Business Administration

Charles Hertzberg, Handicapped Assistance Loans Unit

Richard Lewis, Handicapped Assistance Loans Unit

U.S. Department of Agriculture

Steve Carlson, Food and Nutrition Service, Budget Office

George Dyson, Food and Nutrition Service, Budget Office

U.S. Department of Commerce

Shelby Herman, GNP Price Deflator Section

U.S. Department of Defense

Richard D. Barnett, CHAMPUS Office, Statistics Branch

Valerie Nolan, CHAMPUS Office, Statistics Branch

U.S. Department of Education

Martin Abramson, Ph.D., Office of Special Education

Frank Caracciolo, Rehabilitation Services Administration, Office of Developmental Programs, Special Recreation Projects Unit

Richard Champion, Ph.D. Office of Special Education Division of Innovation and Development

Karen Chauvin; Bureau of Adult, Vocational, and Technical Education

Steve Cohen, Rehabilitation Services Administration

Walter Devins, Rehabilitation Services Administration, Projects with Industry Unit Office of Developmental Programs

Carroll Dexter, Ph.D., Impact Aid Program

Robert Gilmore, Ph.D., Rehabilitation Services Administration, Office of Developmental Programs, Severely Disabled Projects and Demonstrations Unit

Jim Hamilton, Ph.D., Office of Special Education, Division of Research

Jim Johnson, Ph.D., Office of Special Education, Instructional Media Program

Art Kelly, Department of Education, Regional Liaison Unit

Ann Kibler; Bureau of Adult, Vocational, and Technical Education

Kay Little, National Institute of Handicapped Research

Larry Mars, Rehabilitation Services Administration, Office of the Commissioner

Max Mueller, Ph.D., Office of Special Education, former director of the Research Division

Harry Phillips, Ph.D., Congressional Relations Office

Hal Shay, Ph.D., Rehabilitation Services Administration, former director of Training

James Siantz, Ph.D., Office of Special Education, Division of Personnel Preparation

Paul Thompson, Ph.D., Office of Special Education, Severely Handicapped Projects Program

Gloria White, Rehabilitation Services Administration, Budget Office

Bill Wolfe, Office of Special Education, Budget Office

U.S. Department of Health and Human Services

Herman Allen, Division of Vocational Rehabilitation and Special Programs, Office of Disability

Kay Allen, Social Security Administration, Office of Research and Statistics

Rick Beisel, Health Care Financing Administration, Medicaid Statistics Branch, Office of Financial and Actuarial Analysis

Richard Bell, Social Security Administration, Office of Supplemental Security Income

George Bouthilet, Ph.D., President's Committee on Mental Retardation

Matthew Brown, Health Care Financing Administration, Long-Term Care Services Branch

Bob Cormier, Social Security Administration, Office of Research and Statistics

Emmet Dye, Social Security Administration, Office of Family Assistance

Darlene Gurwitz, National Institute of Mental Health, Budget Office

Betsy Hanczaryk, Health Care Financing Administration, Division of State Agency Financial Management

Rudolph Hornmuth, Health Services Administration, Maternal and Child Health Service

Joyce Jackson, Health Care Financing Administration, Medicaid Eligibility Policy Office

Jack Kenyon, Action Agency, Office of Older American Volunteer Programs, chief of Foster Grandparent Program Branch

Douglas Klafein, Office of Human Development Services, Head Start Budget Bureau

Fred Krause, former director of President's Committee on Mental Retardation

Jeff Kunkel, Social Security Administration, Office of the Actuary

Gontran Lamberty, M.D., Maternal and Child Health Service, director of Maternal and Child Health Research Program

Phil Lerner, Social Security Administration, Office of Research and Statistics

Bill Matthews; National Institutes of Health; National Institute of Neurological, Communicative Disorders and Stroke; Budget Office

Steve Meskin, Health Care Financing Administration, Medicaid Cost Estimates Branch

Donald Muse, Health Care Financing Administration, director of Bureau of Data Management and Strategy

Neil Nieman; Social Security Administration; Office of Management, Budget and Personnel

John Nutter, Ph.D., National Institute of Allergy and Infectious Diseases, Program Planning and Evaluation Office

Jim Papai, Health Services Administration, Division of Maternal and Child Health, Office of Training

Penny Pine, Health Care Financing Administration, Bureau of Data Management and Strategy, Division of Information Analysis, Statistical Information Services Unit

Jim Rich, Children's Bureau, Budget Office

Jack Schmulowitz; Social Security Administration; Office of Research, Statistics, and International Policy; Division of Statistics and Analysis

Lois Sparklin, Office of the Assistant Secretary for Management and Budget, Office of Real Facilities Engineering

Aaron Stopak; Social Security Administration; Office of Management, Budget and Personnel

Dave Wood, Health Care Financing Administration, Bureau of Data Management and Strategy, Division of Information Analysis, Statistical Information Services Unit

Jane Zagata, National Institutes of Health, National Institute of Child Health and Human Development, Budget Office

*U.S. Department
of Housing and Urban Development*

Sandy Falconer, Office of Management Information Systems, Direct Loan Branch

U.S. Department of Labor

Bob Rann, Employment and Training Administration, Office of Special National Level Programs, Office of Strategic Planning and Policy Development, Handicapped Projects Coordinator

Nonfederal Respondents

Jack Crosby, Michigan Department of Mental Health, associate director of Finance Division

Carol Dunlap, Electronic Industries Foundation, director of DOL Project

Gary Gesaman, Iowa Department of Human Services, Bureau of Medicaid Services, Long-Term Care Section

Jack Scott, Goodwill Industries of America, director of DOL Projects With Industry Project

Gordon Soloway, Wisconsin Department of Health and Social Services, Nursing Home Unit

Index